# THE LIFE-AFFIRMING MAGIC OF BIRDS

# THE LIFE-AFFIRMING MAGIC OF BIRDS

and the extraordinary
things they can teach us

## CHARLIE BINGHAM

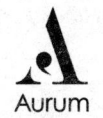

Aurum

# Quarto

First published in hardback in 2025 by Aurum,
an imprint of The Quarto Group
One Triptych Place, London, SE1 9SH
United Kingdom
T (0)20 7700 9000
www.Quarto.com/Aurum

EEA Representation, WTS Tax d.o.o., Žanova ulica 3, 4000 Kranj, Slovenia

Text copyright © 2025 Charlie Bingham
Design © 2025 Quarto
Illustrations © 2025 Luke Western Art LTD

The moral right of Charlie Bingham to be identified as the author of this Work has been asserted by her in accordance with the Copyright, Designs and Patents Act 1988.

All rights reserved.

No part of this publication may be reproduced, stored in a retrieval system, or transmitted, in any form, or by any means, electronic or mechanical, including photocopying, recording or by any information storage and retrieval system, without permission in writing from the publisher.

A catalogue record for this book is available from the British Library.

ISBN: 978-1-83600-225-3
E-book ISBN: 978-1-83600-227-7
Audiobook ISBN: 978-1-83600-620-6

10 9 8 7 6 5 4 3 2 1

Cover artwork by Alison Ingram
Interior artwork by Luke Western Art LTD
Typeset in Bembo by Typo•glyphix, Burton-on-Trent, DE14 3HE

Printed and bound by CPI Group (UK) Ltd, Croydon, CR0 4YY

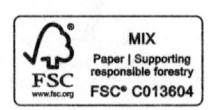

MIX
Paper | Supporting
responsible forestry
FSC® C013604

*See you in the morning,
when the sun is shining,
and the birds are singing.*

# Contents

*Introduction   p1*

**1**
Oystercatcher
Let nature guide you through adversity   *p10*

**2**
Swift
You have the power to change a world   *p34*

**3**
Starling
Look for the unexpected   *p53*

**4**
Peregrine
Learn from those who are there to teach   *p71*

**5**
Swallow
We aren't removed from nature,
we don't own nature, we are nature   *p97*

**6**
Gannet
Our fight or flight response needs a system upgrade   *p116*

**7**
Herring Gull
Nature teaches us the power of resilience   *p138*

**8**
Curlew
Never lose that sense of wonder   *p160*

**9**
Goose
The world can be so much bigger
when you let nature in   *p182*

**10**
Rook
There is beauty in the everyday   *p205*

**11**
Parakeet
Things change, that's guaranteed – it's up to you whether
you choose to change with them   *p219*

**12**
Pigeon
Open your eyes now to the magic
that surrounds you   *p247*

*Special Thanks*   *p264*

# INTRODUCTION

*'Let me be that I am and seek not to alter me.'*
— *Much Ado About Nothing,*
Act 1, Scene 3

It's an interesting reflection on society to think how blinkered we are by our busy lives. We can go about our business without so much as a glance when the tiny robin delivers a crescendo, without looking at the striking rainbow plumage worn by the starling nesting on next door's roof. Despite living in a country which is inhabited by over two hundred different species of bird that breed regularly, I was once guilty of never really paying attention to nature. Actually, that's not true. As a child, I was mad about it. I went everywhere with a bucket or bag specifically for collecting interesting rocks which I would then bring home and decorate with those stick-on earrings from Claire's Accessories for eyes, and then paint patterns with nail polish to make them truly unique works of art. I think my mum still has a shiny blue-painted rock named rather originally, Rocky, from that time, and now, years later, the gravel outside my house is probably 50 per cent rocks and sticks that my own children have collected each time we leave the house. Flower beds in the garden are packed with sticks and stones that they have snuck back from days out, pockets rattling with reminders of explorative days at the beach, and memories that have been created and stored in our minds and hearts. The occasional crab leg making it into my handbag only to be discovered when it starts to whiff. My youngest son once struggled his way down the side of Snowdon, laden with arms full of unusual shaped pieces of Welsh slate that he couldn't possibly live without.

I spent a large portion of my childhood days surrounded by the Yorkshire countryside, monitoring frogspawn in a pond at the side of the local farmer's field and fishing in the ditch for creatures I knew nothing about but found fascinating, nonetheless. I experimented with every recipe for mud pies, deciding my own secret formula was the best, converted the window boxes of my wooden Wendy house into worm farms, and often brought snails into the house to watch them slide along the kitchen surfaces.

As a teenager in rural France, with a forest behind our garden, wild boar were known to roam in the trees, and coypu emerged from the pond to explore the long grass that Dad would only ever get part way through cutting on his sit-on lawnmower. I spent hours with friends, running around the fields, climbing in and out of the pool to escape from the burning summer sun, rescuing insects which had fallen victim to its grip. Now, I am aware of how much we took this for granted, a childhood surrounded by the majesty of nature, and all that entails. Or was it because we are so intrinsically linked to nature that it felt like part of us, rather than something separate to be marvelled at?

The excitement of nature soon disappeared. Much like that belief in childhood fairy tales or the Loch Ness Monster, the magic faded away until getting mud on my new trainers simply wasn't cool and the pleasure of hearing birdsong was

## INTRODUCTION

replaced by keeping up with the trend. Nature no longer existed to me.

People often say they have no interest in birds, but I realised when listening to the author and brilliant naturalist Nick Acheson, speaking on BBC Radio 4 about geese, that everyone has a bird story. I know I probably shouldn't tell you to stop reading my book now, but just for a second, close these pages and think about *your* bird story. What is it? Where was it? How did you feel?

Remember back to a time when you really noticed a bird or interacted with one. Was it a fledgling which fell down your chimney, perhaps? A herring gull swooping down to steal a chip as you promenaded down a busy seafront with friends? You'll have a story. We all have one. You may just have to think hard to find it, but it's there.

As an adult, I can regale you with countless bird stories. And I do, to anyone who happens to make eye contact with me, though sometimes my excitement over the nesting rooks in the school playground gets funny looks from the other mums. And yet when I think back to the time before birds properly entered my life, I have just one story, from when I was fifteen.

Lying on the grass of the family home, my dyed red hair glowed twice as brightly as a freshly painted postbox as I basked in the July sun. A shape dashing above caught my gaze. My bird ID skills were virtually non-existent then, but as the sunlight bounced off the navy plumage, shining like a freshly glazed ceramic work of art, I immediately knew what this was, what I was looking at. A swallow. And suddenly there were five of them, twirling and tumbling in the sky above my head.

## THE LIFE-AFFIRMING MAGIC OF BIRDS

Swallows have always held meaning for Mum and me. Her dad had two swallows tattooed in the space between his thumb and forefinger, and throughout my life, swallows have always seemed to appear when I needed some kind of sign or direction.

That remained my only bird story for another twelve years, until I found myself standing on a muddy shoreline looking out at the Menai Strait in North Wales. We'll deal with that properly later in the book but suffice it to say that it was life changing. That was the moment I became a self-certified bird nerd. In that moment, I noticed a bird that changed everything, that introduced to me a whole new world that was just waiting to be explored. A whole new world that brought a new level of colour, excitement and wonder to my life.

Fast forward from that day on the Menai Strait to Norfolk, where I now live. A significantly different habitat, the North Norfolk coast is bursting with biodiversity and offers up a whole array of species that are now a part of my everyday life. The first time I experienced it, I was overcome, accidentally spotting sand martins which shot in and out of burrows in the cliffs; ruff, with their extravagant plumage during the breeding season, and lapwing, their iridescent bodies still dazzling me to this day, particularly when a bird of prey flies through the crowd, sending them up in a flurry of sparkling flutters like confetti on a day of celebration. That's the magic of nature.

---◊---

I drove my parents mad as a child, switching from one hobby to another like a bee, flitting from one flower to the next, while deciding which stamen might offer the finest pollen.

## INTRODUCTION

I tortured them for hours with piano lessons, jumped to the violin, swore a clarinet was the instrument for me before declaring that, in fact, the cornet my grandad had given me was my true calling. Spoiler alert – it wasn't.

I was lucky that my school offered a wide selection of extra-curricular activities and, excluding the sports clubs, I think I probably tried them all. My mum still has an odd assortment of the remnants of attempted art projects. A rag doll I stitched out of an old tea towel, an egg cup with the face of what I think was eleven-year-old Charlie's attempt at a cat, a purple heart-shaped cushion with 'M U M' awkwardly sewn on to the front, examples of me trying to find an activity that would occupy my mind and keep it engaged.

Nothing changed as I entered adulthood. I've wasted an alarming amount of money on books, craft supplies and online courses, determined to apply myself and learn something new which would soon fade into the back of my mind. My drawers are crammed with half-finished projects. At twenty-six, a diagnosis of ADHD – attention deficit hyperactivity disorder – provided me with a reason for why I had spent my life jumping from one obsession to another, never quite able to settle, and that diagnosis has changed the way I look at myself. It's made me realise that I'm not 'lazy', as I was often told at school. 'Charlie has potential but lacks the ability to apply herself.' Suddenly, I wasn't useless, as I'd previously thought. My life wasn't meaningless. It turns out I am something after all. Neurodivergent. My brain functions in a different way to what's considered the 'norm'. I just needed to find my thing.

Nature.

And more specifically, birds.

Once I reconnected with nature, I couldn't stop. Suddenly, my days spent on the beach came to life with sanderlings, sandpipers, dunlin and turnstones. Birds that had always been there, I just hadn't been looking. The more time I spent searching for them, the more engrossed I became in these fascinating creatures, and the more species seemed to reveal themselves to me.

Since my diagnosis, I'd learnt that some people with ADHD need to have a constant stream of new things to engage the brain, and I realised that all of the other hobbies I had tried previously had not pushed the right buttons for me. Birds are different. They are not static; they're always changing. From the species that come and sample the treats in the garden feeders, to the migrant species which visit from every part of the world, no two birding days are the same. Nothing is guaranteed when you're looking for birds; there's always a surprise. And that is why once I discovered my own bird story, my life began to change.

———◊———

After navigating life as a single parent, my financial situation had taken a nosedive. I found myself suddenly having to claim Universal Credit and use food banks. It was a situation I hadn't foreseen, but once there, it felt impossible to climb out of the black hole my mental health had plummeted to. After finishing my degree as a mature student; I took the step to move to Wales to pursue a masters degree, however, it transpired that a student loan wasn't enough to pay the university fees and also sustain a decent life with my two children. Soaring rental prices and a rising cost of living meant, after careful consideration, that I had to step back

## INTRODUCTION

from education and somehow find a new path, to redirect the trajectory of my life. That, paired with monumental personal loss which sent me into spiralling grief, and I found myself feeling somewhat lost.

But then it changed. I found a bird and that bird somehow showed me a light and a direction. Okay it wasn't as easy as discovering a bird and everything was fine; I wish I could tell you it was that easy. But somehow, and I can't explain why, one bird led to two, and two birds have led to a now neverending curiosity in the world around me that has taught me no matter what's happening in my head, I can go out to my local reserve and nature will help me find a way through. It's realising that I am a tiny part of an unimaginably huge universe that will continue to turn long after my time on Earth is over. Understanding that made me want to thrive again, like a flower who has been waiting for spring. And that's what I did.

So, how does this all relate to this book, you may ask? Well, I'd like to share my experiences with you. To show you how birds can be life changing if you just take the time to look, to wonder. To let them in.

This isn't a bird guide, by any means, and I suppose it isn't a traditional narrative. It's me showing you my journey and my wonder, hoping that you may share it, or learn to. That my own experiences may help you on your way forward through introducing you to the world of birds. Over the next twelve chapters, I intend to share with you a collection of stories about my experiences with some birds around the UK, native and not. And along the way, I hope to introduce you to some of the wonderful 'lessons' that I've learnt from these birds, things which have helped me – and continue to help me – navigate life, death and the world. By showing you this, perhaps you'll see the magic of these birds, too.

In the following pages, I travel from urban locations to mountain peaks in search of these brilliant birds, bringing with me friends who have also had their own unique forays into nature, as well as speaking with individuals who have dedicated their lives to the natural world. But here is the catch you were waiting for. It's not just my journey, it's your journey too. By coming with me on this journey, as I explore some of the wonderful avian species found across the UK, you'll dive headfirst into the natural world.

How will this book work? Well, I'll start with the moment that one bird changed the course of my life in June 2021, and then I'll take you back through a wiggling collection of dated stories from a time when nature wasn't really on my radar at all, all the way through to now. The process may feel like you are being flung around in the TARDIS in an episode of *Doctor Who*, but that's how my journey has been. Writing this book has given me the chance to reflect on a lot of moments in my life where nature has been there and has had an impact on me; I just didn't realise it until I took this time to think about it and write it down. And after writing it down and trying to piece together the somewhat chaotic thoughts that ricochet across my mind, in the same way the call of a bearded tit pings across a reed bed like a vintage pinball machine, it's apparent that nature has been teaching me lessons throughout my whole life. I just didn't realise it.

Birds are a way to engage with nature that is accessible to anyone wanting to experience it and this book will show you how. Anyone can be a birder, if they want to. Anyone. If you are able to use any of your senses (apart from taste,

## INTRODUCTION

you just can't lick a bird), then you can be 'a birder'. If you can hear the beatboxing starling from the tree outside your garden, you can be a birder. If you can see the flash of navy plumage as a swallow circles above you, while you lie on the grass looking up to the sky, you can be a birder. If you can feel the branches of the hedgerows that open their doors to the roosting flock of sparrows each night, then you can be a birder. If you can smell the rich scent of flora coming to life in spring, feeding the countless species that make their way to spend summers here with us, then guess what, you can be a birder. These are just a few examples, but they show, if you want to, that you can experience the wonder birds bring, too.

There is a community of brilliant bird nerds out there just waiting to welcome you with open arms, who couldn't give a flying phalarope if you know your pink feet from your beans, your tits from your boobies – and we are going to meet some of them in this book. So, without further ado, let's turn the key and fly through the magical gateway and learn how to see the world through a new lens.

And let's discover your bird story.

# 1
# OYSTERCATCHER

*'Why then the world's mine oyster,
Which I with sword will open.'*
– The Merry Wives of Windsor,
Act 2, Scene 2

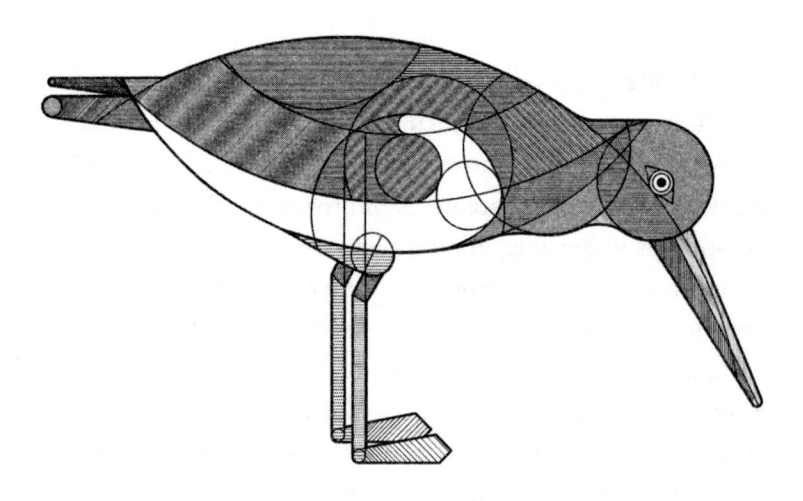

**Let nature guide you through adversity**

Oystercatchers.

Wading birds, iconic stars of coastal landscapes, filling the air with their high-pitched calls which seem to echo, carried by the light ocean breeze. Their song seems to stand out in a soundscape, unique and bold.

An oystercatcher was the bird who changed it all for me, who captured my curiosity and showed me that there was more to life than the turbulence in my own head. It taught me that life is fleeting, and we should say yes to opportunity, seizing the moment – *carpe diem*, to quote that old cliché. This chapter isn't going to be just about oystercatchers though. It's about welcoming birds into our lives and using them as a gateway to the vast natural world that turns around us and as a way to bring light into darkness, of feeling less alone at those difficult points in our lives.

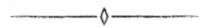

---

It's June 2021 and I'm on the beach looking out across the Menai Strait in North Wales.

My bare feet slid against the velvety silt as the tide flowed in and out like a deep breath. Each time, it pulled the earth away from under me, allowing me to sink further. Small stones brushed against my toes and the rough sand, mixed into the mud, grated along my skin.

Being barefoot on a cold beach is a sensory experience like no other. Type 'the benefits of barefoot walking' into a Google search and you will be met with a confusing array of mixed messages. Some researchers claim it's detrimental to your body and will result in fallen arches. Other sources cite the benefits of allowing your skin to connect with the ground, claiming it improves blood flow, eases insomnia and even boosts cardiovascular health. Either way, as my feet were engulfed by the freezing sea, each new texture brought me closer to the earth and took me further away from the thoughts racing in my mind.

Closing my eyes, I allowed the soft breeze to fill my nostrils. The momentary silence was broken by the delighted cheers of my two young children behind me, who were creating piles of shingle to demolish with their toy trucks. I looked up to my right at the giant that towered above, the walls of Caernarfon Castle, built seven hundred years ago by Edward I as a fortress to defend against potential assault.

A slight movement caught my attention.

Glancing over, I expected to see my eldest child collecting salty water in a bottle to add to the shingle sculpture they were constructing. Instead, a bird, slightly smaller than a crow, stood about 8 metres away. It seemed to be looking into the distance, just as I'd been, perhaps sensing a disturbance in the force and feeling the need to remain vigilant. My fellow sea gazer was a sight to behold: a perfect black plumage covered its head, flowing across its back and wings. Some scraggly feathers stuck up awkwardly, as if awaiting preening. Its chest and belly were, in contrast, a pure white. I remember wondering how could it remain so clean when my own skin was coated in dried pale brown mud.

The bird's beak was long and thin, deep orange in colour with a yellow tip. It reminded me of a bright pair of tweezers I had sitting on the side of the downstairs bathroom sink at home. Carefully designed to tease its prey from their shells like peeling an awkward splinter from under the skin of your finger. And standing out on its black head, like Jupiter against a clear night sky, was one red eye. Long pink legs extended from its black and white body and I watched it wading through the mud in the direction of the others similarly so strikingly dressed. Something about them made me think of the penguin from *Wallace and Gromit*. As the bird disappeared into the flock which picked their way through the silt, my ears tuned into their sound, their loud *'peep peep'*-ing carrying across the beach to where I stood watching.

I'd never seen a bird like this before, and for the first time since I lost the sense of magic in nature, curiosity got the better of me. Breaking my promise to have a technology-free afternoon, I pulled out my phone and typed the following phrase:

*black and white bird at the beach going peep peep*

Admitting that this was my method for identifying my first bird used to cause me some embarrassment, but I have used this technique plentiful times now including most recently to identify a redwing:

*small bird with a red wing*

To my surprise, the first Google search result was an exact match to the birds wading along the shallows in front of me.

*Oystercatcher*

It may sound dramatic but seeing that one bird changed my life. It opened up a new world for me, one to which I had temporarily lost the key. Wildlife cameraman and *Strictly Come Dancing* champion Hamza Yassin once said to me that he saw birds as a gateway to nature. That is exactly what that oystercatcher meant to me. That one bird opened the door to nature and to a new way of thinking about my life, how I dealt with things and navigated the world.

So, there you have it: that is the moment I became a self-certified bird nerd.

But while I had found 'my thing', I still had a way to go to fully immerse myself in this pastime. I soon discovered that there were many hurdles in place. From financial constraints and safety while spending time in nature, to facing the gatekeepers who seem to present the terms and conditions for participating in it, I found all of these barriers are surmountable if we choose to take the power into our hands.

———◊———

A text comes through to my phone, causing the whole sofa to vibrate aggressively. It's from Connor, my kid's dad, and I can see he has sent a video, which is unusual. We chat still, but usually only about the kids so I can't think what it could possibly be.

'What the hell is this and why is it doing that, it's been going on for hours?' his text reads.

Opening up the video to full screen, I smile as I hear that familiar 'peep peep' sound coming loudly from my phone speaker. An oystercatcher is standing proudly on the rooftop opposite his house and shouting its song across the street. Connor lives about an hour inland from me, so it seems weird to think of the bird being so far away from the sea. But then I remember something I read about them nesting on rooftops, using them as a proxy for the shingle beaches that they would naturally lay their eggs on, so I suppose this isn't really that unusual.

In normal circumstances, oystercatchers are birds of shorelines and tidal estuaries, sometimes breeding in unexpected places. Along the Norfolk coast, I often watch them wandering up and down the sandy beaches, weaving in and out of groups of walkers and taking flight as their dogs bound happily in and out of the sea. As their name suggests, they are partial to an oyster or two, their elongated bill providing the perfect tool for handling this kind of prey. In fact, some individuals have shorter bills which they use to hammer open their meals, while others have longer, pointier bills which they can use to carefully prise open treats. They don't eat just oysters, though, and can be found snacking on other bivalves like cockles and mussels.

If you ever find yourself in the company of oystercatchers, sit down on the sand for a while and watch them as they navigate their way up the coastline sampling the buffet available to them. Listen out for the distinctive *'peep peep'* sound, which is remarkably loud for a bird no bigger than a duck! Typically, during the spring and summer months, they will be guarding their nests, which they create out in the open, and where they lay two to three eggs that are perfectly camouflaged by the shingle and vegetation surrounding them. Except when they're nesting on rooftops in urban areas.

Our impact on the natural world, particularly urbanisation, has caused a massive decline in biodiversity. The 2023 *State of Nature Report* detailed that some 43 per cent of birds in the UK are in population decline, but there is evidence to suggest that urban environments can play a role in protecting threatened species, including, perhaps surprisingly, oystercatchers. A 2024 paper by a group of German scientists found that the reproductive success in those birds nesting on flat rooftops was high. They concluded that this was likely the rooftop location provided safety from predators, and suggested that this knowledge, and the potentially positive impact on a species forced to live in an ever-growing urban world, should be taken into consideration when planning and managing new developments. If only it were as easy to get people to adapt, hey?

While I'm still not sure I would call myself a 'birder' and I don't think I know enough to be called a 'naturalist', I have a strong interest and curiosity. My route to reconnection with nature has been a very personal journey that has, at times, been turbulent and, at times, acted as therapy. It's something that has been there for me at my darkest moments, and a learning curve – something that, in hindsight, I could have perhaps benefited from at the hardest points in my life, those times when I felt most bereft or alone, if I'd only realised how beneficial time spent with nature, with birds, was for me.

There have been two major losses in my life. They happened a few years apart, when I was at very different points on my journey. I want to reflect on how nature could have helped me, and how nature did help me, and by doing so, I hope it can help you too if the time comes where you feel like you're floundering in the dark. They say that the only things certain in life are death and taxes, and while I'm not sure connecting with nature can help with your tax return, when dealing with death, that's a different story.

———◊———

I was twenty-two and had a five-week-old baby boy. My whole world had been redefined after I'd spent the couple of years since finishing a musical theatre college course, flitting from situation to situation, with little direction. Ambition, yes, but nowhere to focus it, so I jumped from job to job. A year as a dental nurse, a season as a Center Parcs high ropes and abseiling instructor, a few months in a furniture factory working in the complaints department. Unfulfilled, confused, and now I had a whole new human to try and figure out how to raise. Looking back at that time, I feel like I was only a baby myself. So young and underprepared, about to embark on a journey with my son where we would learn together, navigating life's highs and lows, getting to know each other as well as getting to know ourselves for the first time.

Every parent is a new parent once. Each experience is the first once. The first nappy change, the first bump on the head, the first emotional toddler explosion in the middle of Asda, the first day of school, the first homework, the first time they have a disagreement with a friend, the first time they experience heartbreak. I think people, myself included, forget that parents are learning too. My mum didn't know what she was doing when she had me. Like me, everything was new to her: she'd never experienced holding my hand while I took my first steps; she'd never taken me for my first day of school and known what it was to walk away while I screamed the place down. She'd never experienced raising a teenage girl until I became one. She couldn't have known what it would be like to help twenty-something me through an unplanned pregnancy until it happened. And she'd never really thought about the role, the very vital role, she might play in raising her grandsons, in helping me shape them. She'd never done or thought about any of these things, and yet she did each of them with unconditional love, endless commitment and support. She raised me, a daughter, despite never having done so before and, as clichéd as it sounds, she gave me the world, and still does, with no expectation. Each experience between a parent and child is a new one, so we need to cut each other some slack. But at this point I didn't think about all this, just the enormity of being a young mother with a baby.

## THE LIFE-AFFIRMING MAGIC OF BIRDS

My mum had a younger brother, John. He didn't realise it, but he was brilliant. And a total arse, to be honest. Sarcastic, with a really dry sense of humour, a light Scouse accent with a unique tone to his voice that I can still hear if I try hard enough. 'G-o-d!' he'd shout, elongating the vowel with passion, at the TV, when my grandma would watch *The X Factor*. 'Load of shite.' He didn't say much, but he was one of those silent observers who occasionally would come out with the best lines that would crack everyone up while he remained stony-faced.

John, unfortunately, had been the victim of a series of events that resulted in him turning to alcohol. He was a functioning alcoholic. So functioning that those closest to him didn't realise it. He was a medical professional and understood perfectly what was happening to his body, yet was able to conceal it with plausible excuses. By the time my mum, who is also from a medical background, realised what her brother had been dealing with alone, it was too late and his mind was made up. He didn't want help; he knew what he was doing and understood perfectly the consequences.

'I'm going up to John tonight, I think it's really serious,' my mum's text flashed on my phone as I made up the final bottle of the evening for baby Jack, who was bouncing in his chair next to my border collie. In the absence of a sheep to herd, Mac had taken it upon himself to provide private security for the baby and did so with extreme dedication and love.

I called Mum back but she didn't answer as she was driving, it turned out. Somehow I knew this was it. I think I'd actually known the last time I'd seen John. He'd driven my grandma down to visit me when I was heavily pregnant and had spent the whole visit pacing, sweating, shaking, vomiting in the toilet. He blamed a new medication – in reality he'd forced himself to go cold turkey so that he could see me one last time. He knew. As he handed me £100 to get a 3D-baby scan done, kissed me on the head and told me he loved me for the first time in my life, I knew, too. This would be the last time I'd see him.

'Go to bed, sleep while the baby sleeps, I'll let you know if anything happens,' a text came through a couple of hours later.

When the landline rang in the living room, I looked at the time, 6 a.m., and got out of the bed, leaving Connor, Jack's dad, half-asleep with Jack, who was awake in his Moses basket, peacefully examining the farm animal mobile above his head. Moving quickly across the bungalow's narrow hallway to the living room, I stood by the phone, my hand hovering over the receiver until it clicked to the answering machine. I just wanted to exist in a world where John was still alive for a moment longer, wanted to live in a universe where he was still shouting at the telly, at *The X Factor* or watching reruns of *The Royle Family*.

Just a few moments longer.

I steadied myself and, without listening to the message, redialled the number I knew by heart, moving back to the bedroom where Connor was now sat up in bed to see what was going on. My mum answered immediately. I heard the tears through the words she spoke with the strength that she has always shown. I didn't say anything, I didn't need to, instead taking a deep breath while I leaned back against the doorway, as memories flashed through my mind.

## THE LIFE-AFFIRMING MAGIC OF BIRDS

Sitting on a wooden box in John's music room with an acoustic guitar in my hand, him getting stressed and me laughing at him as he tried to teach me the opening chords to 'Wonderwall'.

A pub quiz, him shouting out the answers so the whole pub kept tutting at him while he smirked having achieved the desired reaction.

His stupid ringtone, the *Z-Cars*' theme: he was an Evertonian.

That ridiculous tattoo of a Beatles 'Yellow Submarine' character he had on his leg.

Me, hiding in the spare room at John and my grandma's house, aged sixteen, sobbing over my first experience of heartbreak and John walking up the stairs and silently hugging me.

I never told him, never expressed how I felt, never let him know how important he was to me. A leading figure in my life, now gone.

'I'll let everyone know,' I told my mum.

I was a mum now, it was my job to lead, to be strong for the family and to take on that protective role. This is what I told myself, a way to avoid feeling feelings that didn't want to be felt. Feelings that, in fact, I still haven't felt. I shed the occasional tear when I hear an Oasis song, John's favourite band, or when I think about big life events that he has missed, but I've never come to terms with it. In fact, this is the first time I've ever put these feelings out into the world. I have had no way of processing these feelings, no place of solace and no outlet for the emotions.

Then came Clyde, my cousin.

He was incredible. I know everyone says that, but really, he was the personification of light. He illuminated every room he entered with his smile and his vibrant energy. He had formed an extra special relationship with Jack and showered him with love. Jack loved his 'Jazzy Clyde', a name we still aren't sure where the three-year-old plucked it from, but it suited and it stuck. Clyde did everything for everyone. He was a musician, a singer and an entertainer, literally the sunrise in all of our lives.

In 2021, Covid raged through the world. We had been released from lockdown and were living in Wales. I had taken the kids camping at Shell Island, a beautiful, peaceful and isolated campsite in North Wales. I got a little bit of a signal and saw I had a message from Clyde.

'Hi babes, I'm in ICU with Covid, been here for 4 days total miracle drugs, I'm so blessed and can't believe how far I've come, gonna smash it don't worry xx.'

'What? Okay, but you're on the mend, right?' I replied, shaking slightly.

'Yes, they have performed small miracles. I can't believe it, sats dropped to 30 but now up to 73.'

'Okay, message or call me anytime, we will see you soon,' I texted back, with positive hope.

'Love u all so much, can't wait to meet up soon, it's been too long.'

That was to be the last message I ever received.

Did he know?

That night, I woke up to my pillow vibrating with my cousin Rachael's name flashing on the screen. 'Clyde isn't good babe, we are all at the hospital. I'll let you know what happens.'

I looked at Jack and prayed that his Jazzy Clyde pulled through this, that I wouldn't have to tell him bad news.

The morning came with no news and I went through the whole day feigning a smile for my boys, as parents do, the worry piling up inside me.

That evening, as the sun was getting ready to set, we walked down to the beach and I sat down on a flat rock while the kids ploughed their way on to the sand, bare feet sliding through the shallow water that lapped over their feet. My phone rang and I saw Rachael's name flash up again. 'This is it,' I thought. 'Clyde's gone.'

I took the call, looking at the view, the phone to my ear even after she'd hung up. My boys' laughter reached me and I landed back on Earth. Tears began to pool in my eyes, and I stared out across the sea at the mountain range which lies across the water. The sky was streaked with fiery oranges and reds, lighting up peaks of the mountains and making them glow like something out of a fantasy novel.

'Peep peep. Peep peep.' The birdsong caught my attention.

An oystercatcher landed on the shore near my children and began wading up and down on the hunt for an evening meal. The steel-coloured waves gently touched the bird's pointed feet as it stuck its beak into the sand, foraging for its next tasty morsel. Each gentle footstep brought glistening droplets of salty water that scattered on to the sand, leaving no trace except the memory of what once was. The bird took flight suddenly and sent an echoey sound across the still air as it flew over my head and away. I wondered what the world must look like from up there. What would a bird's eye view of the scene I was part of look like? The bird didn't feel my grief, didn't know that my insides were writhing as

I fought to retain a sense of normality for my children still playing in the sand, unaware. My world had stopped and yet the rest of the world was turning.

As I watched that oystercatcher, though, I felt a weird sense of peace descend. The sun setting in front of me felt like a metaphor, like Clyde saying a final goodbye, the brightest star setting on his journey. Glancing down, I spotted something carved into the rocks where I sat. Peering at it, I saw it was a simple smiling face. A cheeky smile that told a story, I hadn't noticed it before. A tear fell, then another, and my boys, seeming to sense something was wrong, ran over to me, both putting their arms around my neck.

'Is it my Jazzy Clyde, Mummy?' Jack asked.

'Yes, baby.' I never lie to my children or sugarcoat things. 'But we're going to be okay.'

'I know,' he replied simply, holding on tight as we watched the oystercatcher take flight, spooked by an unseen source.

Two losses, two very different experiences.

You could argue that my differing response to these two horrific events was just situational. When John died, it was my first real adult experience of death. I was dealing with the aftermath of a tricky childbirth and navigating my new life as a parent. But I know in my heart that I dealt with Clyde's death in a different way – because of nature. My connection with it, with that bird, meant I had a space to channel my grief, and something there to make me realise that I wasn't alone in this feeling.

Grief is something we will all experience in our lives, but we will all experience it in our own ways. It's something we all unfortunately experience, yet we rarely discuss it in the West, as though it is some kind of taboo subject that must be censored. When John died, I felt alone with my feelings, wondering how on earth I was going to keep on moving. Yet when Clyde died, the oystercatcher, the sunset, the smiling face carved on to the rock, they all made me feel like I was part of something bigger. The sunset taught me that, while the sun might have set on his life, the sun will rise again, as will the beautiful memories I have of Clyde. The oystercatcher taught me about continuity. That by allowing myself to consider the continuity of nature in the face of such adversity, maybe, just maybe, as I am a part of nature, too, I could carry on.

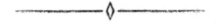

---

It's March 2024. The train passes the Emirates Stadium and I snap a blurred picture as we speed past. Jack is an Arsenal supporter, much to the horror of my dad, a diehard Spurs fan. I'll show him the photo later. Megan Shersby is sitting next to me, a writer, butterfly lover and another all-round nature lover. I haven't actually known Megan that long, but we seem to have settled into one of these effortless friendships. A friendship with no requirements or expectations, just easy. We are on our way to Hampstead Heath to meet Rory Dimond, entomologist and super knowledgeable nature wizard, and Ryan Dalton, nature podcaster extraordinaire, comedian and, like me, someone who somehow manages to find the joy and magic in the everyday. We arrive at Gospel Oak Station where Rory, Ryan and Ryan's dog, Riley, are waiting for us. Megan and I are late, like *really* late, but ultimately that was to be expected. I'm starving as always so we stop off at a tiny café and grab some cheese toasties, cheddar oozing out of doorstep slices of freshly made bread, and as we step on to the leaf-strewn path of Hampstead

Heath, London fades into the background, replaced by the soothing sounds of nature. The air is crisp and cool, carrying with it the promise of spring, and I can't help but feel a sense of anticipation as I embark on this walk. I've wanted to visit Hampstead Heath for years, and I'm not sure why I've never been. I think it's probably anxiety I've built up in my head about getting here. I've only recently got to grips with the city's public transport system, and as I've discovered today, it's really not that hard.

We meander along the winding trails, our conversation flowing as we catch up on each other's lives. All of us keep getting distracted by the smallest things. A dandelion with a bee sitting on top of it, a kestrel hovering overhead, parakeets blending in with the kites being flown by children in the breeze, their streaming tail feathers making them look like part of the sky parade.

'Look at that pigeon, my favourite bird!' I point at a woodpigeon which is foraging in a patch of long grass.

'Bloody pigeon', Ryan replies in jest.

As we get to the top of the hill we have been wandering up, Riley the dog trying to drag a huge branch behind us, my breath is momentarily taken from my lungs as I finally see the view that I've been wanting to see for so long now. I was worried it would be like one of those Instagram reels you see, the panorama you come for vs the panorama you get, followed by some disappointing music and grim reality. But, as I look out at the London skyline, I feel like I could stay here forever.

I feel like I'm on top of the world looking down, a silent observer watching city life from up here in my natural haven.

I stand for a while, lost in the moment, and when I turn around, I am greeted by my three friends, standing, arms folded, waiting patiently for me. When I rejoin the group, Rory asks, 'Have you ever seen a mandarin duck?' I shake my head. To be quite honest, I'm not sure what a mandarin duck is, so in the name of exploration and discovery, we follow him as he weaves his way through the heath.

Ryan diverts us through a woodland, directing us to the wildlife hidden within. 'Do you want to see a baby newt?' We all nod in agreement. This is my idea of a very nice day out.

Ryan and Riley take us to a specific log that they have clearly visited many times before. He gently squats down, rolling it. We all peer in to see what he sees and, sure enough, two baby newts are sheltering beneath it. I try to imagine things from their point of view, four giants (five if you count the dog) staring down at them from above. Imagine someone lifting the roof off your house and looking in!

If you haven't tried it, though, log lifting is addictive. Next time you're out for a walk and you spot a good mossy log that looks like it's been there for a while, trust the process. Go and lift it up or roll it over and have a sneaky look at what's underneath. Often, you'll find woodlice scurrying about, sometimes little millipedes all curled up in a tight coil, bright orange centipedes writhing in the earth, and if you're really lucky, you'll get a treat like a newt or a slow-worm. You may feel like you look a bit mad the first couple of times, but after a while, curiosity takes over. I can't walk past a good log without doing this and you quickly get to know which logs are the juiciest, with the most potential treasure lurking underneath. Just please, if you're going to partake in this cool new hobby, remember to put the log back. How would you feel if someone lifted your house and shifted it a couple of feet away?

Once we've replaced the log, we head off to find these mandarins. My curiosity grows as we approach a large pond. 'There they are,' Rory points.

'Woah!' I exclaim with genuine surprise. 'It's like if one of my kids coloured in a picture of a duck, with no knowledge about what a duck looks like.'

The duck that has caught me off guard is a male mandarin duck. He is a kaleidoscope of colour as he glides across the pond. His head is crowned in a tiara of orange and greens, iridescent feathers glistening like jewels. Moving down his neck, I spot shades of emerald and purple, a creamy white breast and thick black stripes acting as borders between all of the colours, like some kind of modern art piece you might see in the Tate Gallery.

'How cool is that?' the genuine awe in my voice unmistakable. Once again, I am taken aback by the sheer diversity of nature. This bird, like a patchwork quilt in front of my eyes, like the oystercatcher, gives me just another small, momentary glimpse into a vast and vibrant world and makes me want to dive even further in.

The mandarin duck was like a gateway that opened our day up into much more than a quest to find one duck. The mandarin turned our day into a huge adventure, one that enabled us to explore the plants, insects and even reptiles of London. Although the goal was to see the bird, it's impossible to ignore everything else that came with it. There's just so much to see and it's all so incredible and complex.

Once you get into nature, there's no going back. I just love that every time I leave the house, I spot a new cool beetle, hear a bird I've never seen before or spot an unknown flower sprouting through the cracks in the pavement. It's bloody brilliant.

A huge magnolia tree is in full bloom, large white petals drooping slightly. These flowers only last a few weeks, but they certainly make their time with us worthwhile. This specimen is providing a backdrop for a lot of photos, people posing in front of the magnificent feature for their latest Instagram post. I wonder if everyone realises they are, in that moment, connecting with nature. They recognise the beauty and want to capture it. Many of them will then go about their day without a second thought, but I'll hold on to the fact: the connection there.

I saw a video recently about foraging, something I've never trusted myself to do. It said that these leathery magnolia flowers are edible. I was all up for trying it, until I Googled it (safety first) and saw there is more than one type of magnolia and they're not all edible. I didn't bother to research further – like I said, I don't trust myself, I don't think I'm the foraging sort.

Megan grabs a handful of hawthorn leaves off a bush and shoves a couple into my hand, putting the rest in her mouth. Megan *is* the foraging sort. She reminds me of a lecturer I had at the University of York who has sadly passed away now, Don Henderson. An absolute legend in the field of archaeology, but perhaps known to friends for the incredible shapes he would throw on the dance floor at any event. He was a forager. I remember watching him walk through the courtyard of King's Manor, the home of York archaeology, one day, his arms full of books. He stopped at a tree and, like a giraffe, outstretched his neck and bit a few of the fresh green leaves off the branches, chomping away. A beautiful soul connected to his surroundings.

'God it's like eating grass. What's the point?' I ask Megan in mild confusion. Why would she waste energy chewing on these tiny leaves.

'A light snack,' she shrugs. She is my kind of weird.

'Right, pub?' I suggest. The drizzle is starting to trickle down my neck and I don't have a raincoat with me.

I look around as we walk, thinking about all of the people who are on the Heath. There are loads of them. Some tourists are taking selfies, a woman walking a baby Great Dane called Michael who is the size of a small horse and is currently terrorising an elderly dachshund. Families sit on blankets with components that once made up picnics strewn around them. A couple are on a bench in heated discussion. These people could be anywhere and yet they chose to be here today. Are they all, like me, seeking solace from a busy city environment? Or is it just somewhere to go for a cheap day out? Why do humans seem to naturally flock to these green spaces? Is it some innate desire to connect with something that we instinctively know we belong in? Whatever the reason, I'm glad I am sharing this moment with these three people who just get it.

Sitting down in the pub, a parakeet screeches overhead, welcoming us and letting us know it's there. 'Thank you, guys, honestly, I've had the best day,' I say with genuine gratitude.

I'm glad I got to share Hampstead Heath with them. For a few hours, we've been adventurers, uncovering an undiscovered wilderness waiting to be explored. That's the feeling I want every day. That is what I've got since reconnecting with nature. That's the reward.

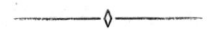

———◊———

June 2024 and I'm in Dinorwic. It's a strange place. One of those places with a really odd 'vibe'. It's an abandoned slate quarry set high above the popular North Wales hiking destination, Llanberis. A two-mile drive up a winding, single track path, which admittedly feels more like ten miles once you've reversed downhill several times to allow vans and other large 'not to be argued with' vehicles past, and you will find yourself at an obvious parking spot, flanked by towering mountainside littered in discarded slate.

After leaving the comfort of the car, I prise the Nintendo Switch out of each of my children's hands and assemble them by the boot to zip them into coats which will protect them from the June drizzle. We are in that weird stage of early summer. You know, when it's meant to be getting warmer, but instead I'm shivering against the low temperature that engulfs us. I'm not sure what I expected from a mountain in North Wales.

We begin the short walk to the quarry site ready to explore and soon we are immersed in a grey scene. Everywhere we look, the floor, the thick walls, the abandoned buildings, a monochrome landscape. The place just feels different. Despite the groups of people, families chattering about their day so far, toddlers running ahead of worried parents, a white fluffy Samoyed dragging his owner back towards the car park, the air is still.

We are heading for a small cave today which leads to a dramatic drop and a small waterfall which constantly trickles against the rock. As we scramble up a narrow path, I look down at a bright blue pool below us, threatening to pull us in with one wrong move. My youngest son, George, stops and has a momentary panic as he, too, looks down into the sky blue pool. 'I can't swim, Mummy. What if I fall?' But after some words of encouragement from me, and a more brutal 'You're halfway there now. You either live here forever or carry on, that's your choice,' from his supportive older brother, we emerge victorious at the entrance to the cave.

I hear a weird noise in the sky above us and immediately look up to try and identify it. It's a bird, of course, but it sounds like an airborne dog has an annoying squeaky toy and is chomping down on it as they fly. I recognise the call, but being one to doubt myself, I can't be sure. I whip out my phone and open the Merlin birdsong app as two black shapes soar into view and tumble behind the adjacent mountainside, disappearing into the slate-filled landscape.

The app brings up 'red billed chough', as I suspected. I've seen these black corvids in Wales before, their blood red bills unmistakable against the Anglesey clifftops, but I'm not convinced I'm seeing them up a mountain, miles away from their typical coastal homes. I text a birdy group chat I'm part of and ask, 'Chough, up a mountain in Wales, am I going mad?' To my surprise, a resounding 'yes you probably have gone mad but also yes it will have been chough' flashes up on my phone screen, and I feel honoured that two endangered birds have decided to share my hike with me today.

I know this chapter is meant to be about oystercatchers, but really, as you've just found out, it's about so much more. Rediscovering nature has opened up my eyes to the things around me, in the pavements and in the forests and mountaintops. It's about life, and the ups and downs that go with it, and how, since rediscovering my connection to nature, things that might once have broken me have become easier to deal with. I feel lighter when I step outside and see another sunrise. I feel energised when I watch a burning sunset knowing (hoping) that it means I get a chance to do this life thing for another day. And that's what this chapter is really about. It's dedicated to the huge variety of opportunities we have every single day to notice nature and the power that nature has to guide us through adversity, if we let it into our lives. Whether it be an oystercatcher on a roundabout on our way into work, or a rare bird up a Welsh mountain, it's all around us.

Take a chiffchaff, for example. A bird that I frequently hear on the Norfolk coast throughout the summer, but which I have also heard in a Welsh mountain town, and in a busy Asda car park in the middle Liverpool. Nature doesn't have to be remote and wild to be spectacular; it's always there, and by learning to notice what is around us, we open ourselves up to a whole world that moves around us as we go about our business, filling up our cars, grabbing a coffee on the way to work or jogging through the park.

Our worlds may stop, but nature stops for no one. I know I bang on about going outside and spotting something new, but it really is that simple. Yet, it's not a cure-all solution. I still feel the burning ache of emptiness and longing when I think about the two men who were taken away from us before we were ready, but I have used nature as an outlet for my grief. The coconut aroma of gorse on a sunny day, the call of a swift as it screams past my house, the baby pigeon with a really wonky beak that is staring through my window as I write, they all remind me that there is still joy out there.

Look outside now, begin that journey down the rabbit hole and let curiosity take hold. Let it lead you through each day, starting now. You may find your oystercatcher. You may find a moment of joy.

# 2
# SWIFT

*'Swift as a shadow, short as any dream,
Brief as the lightning in the collied night.'*
*– A Midsummer Night's Dream,*
Act 1, Scene 1

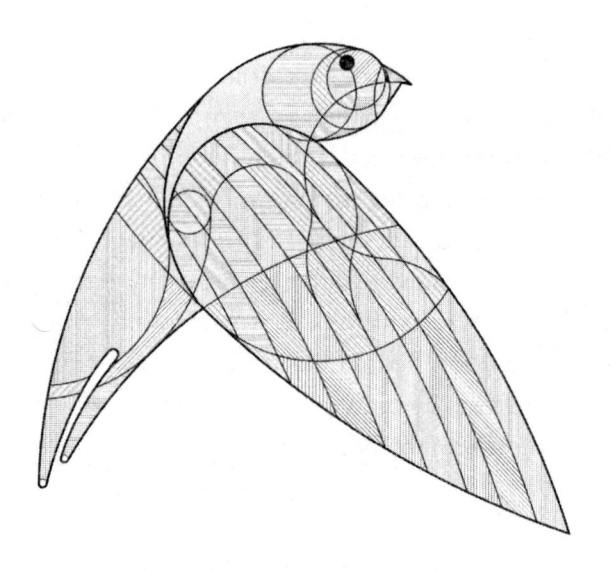

**You have the power to change a world**

If you've ever looked up to the sky as a swirl of screeching swifts gather above you, then you'll know how enchanting, how captivating they are. The swift had a lesson to teach me. They taught me my actions can have a powerful effect on a world, perhaps not the whole world but someone's world. And maybe that's enough to make a change. Let me explain.

# SWIFT

A couple of years ago, if you had told me that one day my thoughts would be consumed by the arrival of a single species of bird to the UK skies, I would have suggested you didn't know me very well at all. If you'd said, one day soon, as the end of April approaches, you will be frustrated as you wait to hear their familiar screech as they fill the air above you, I would have laughed. In fact, a few years ago I don't think I had ever really heard of a swift. Okay, maybe I had heard of them, but I couldn't have pulled one out of a line up. Now I find myself daydreaming as I sit at my laptop, wondering what stage in their journey they are at, as my now old friends make their way from sub-Saharan Africa to spend their summer filling the air above my Norfolk garden with their screaming calls. It's hard to believe that I spent so many years of my life unaware of these birds who travel thousands of miles just to be with us every year. How could I never have noticed them, heard them, felt their presence in my life? My eyes and ears are now pulled upwards at every sight and sound in the sky in the hope that it might be them at last.

---

It's May 2024 and I find myself, once again, standing in the kitchen on autopilot, loading chicken and cheese into wraps and packing Quavers and Fruit Shoots into lunch boxes while the kids eat their toast at a rate of one bite every ten minutes in the living room. I can hear the unmistakable sound of Ali A, a popular British YouTuber, blasting from the television on the wall, no doubt reacting to supposedly satisfying videos of people slicing cake, popping water balloons and colouring neatly in the lines. Things that, to me, are just normal occurrences, but to my children, Jack and George, who would probably spend a lifetime watching these videos given the chance, are 'sick', 'mad skills'.

I'm summoning the energy to begin the usual routine of telling them, once again, to hurry up because they only have ten minutes. Brush your teeth, get your shoes on, get your school bag. Despite now having done this every weekday for the last five years, we still must perform this charade. *Every. Single. Morning.*

Upon entering the room, I find that Ali A is in fact reacting to a video of a woman dipping her ice cream in sand and eating it. At this point, I'm not even going to question it, instead, I pick up the remote and turn the TV off to be met with cries of outrage from the captivated audience.

8.20 a.m. 'You have ten minutes. Brush your teeth, get your bag, put your water in your bag and let's go' I say.

'*I. AM.* Why do you always have to repeat that every single morning?' my eight-year-old, Jack, throws back at me, while remaining motionless on the sofa and staring at the black TV screen. As a brief respite before continuing the script, I perch on the edge of the sofa and open the site formerly known as Twitter on my phone, and see a post from fellow bird nerd and author Lev Parikian.

Lev is a famed swift lover and his words, 'it's zero seconds until the swifts get back, stand down everyone', remind me that it could be anytime now. I had almost forgotten that they should be here soon; consumed in the stress of daily life, my mind still sometimes wanders away from the occurrences outside my window and I find myself entrenched in my own thoughts. But Lev has pulled me back out momentarily and reminded me that, whatever is going on with my life, the natural world will continue to turn. It humbles me, and for a moment the morning routine of trying to get the children out of the door doesn't seem to be so huge. Swifts will at this very moment be arriving after their long-haul flight to fill the skies once again. Would you believe me if I said that after leaving the nest, young swifts spend around the first three years of their lives 'on the wing'? Well, it's true. These weirdly unique birds do, in fact, spend their entire lives, except for a brief nesting period each year, airborne. They're so well suited to a life in the sky, and look totally awkward if you ever see a video of them crawling on the ground, with their tiny legs and feet. They move, on the ground at least, in the same way a bat would, like they're not meant to be there. On the rare occasion that they land, they cling like a gargoyle might, expertly carved into the walls of a cathedral, with their stone-coloured feathers. There are over one hundred species of swifts across the world, and the ones that come to breed in the UK have one of the longest migration journeys of any bird, covering around 14,000 miles each year. I recently read that, if the average swift lives for twenty years, and they are in constant flight (can you imagine flying for twenty years?), scientists predict that they could accumulate around four million air miles in their lives. That's the equivalent of flying around the world 160 times or flying to the moon and back eight times. These birds will fly through the airspaces of twenty-five countries, through storms and blinding sunshine to reach their destinations each year. The more I think about it, the more in awe I am at these feathered gargoyles.

They are aerial feeders, meaning they feed by snatching insects out of the sky as they whizz past them at speeds of up to 69 miles per hour, the fastest recorded species of a bird in level flight. If that's not impressive enough, swifts have been recorded flying over 18,700 feet, as high as some Himalayan peaks. They've evolved a more efficient breathing system, known as a 'uniflow respiratory system', to allow them to fly at great heights where the air is thinner as if they're floating towards the stars. Ethereal and magical beings (though I'm sure an ornithologist would tell you it's a bit more complicated than that).

Swifts belong to a group called *apodiformes*, which include hummingbirds. They share a peculiar wing structure that allows them to be in perpetual flight, and weak feet. Fossil evidence suggests that swifts diverged from the last common ancestor they share with hummingbirds on their evolutionary tree between forty and fifty million years ago. Over time, swifts adapted to their aerial lifestyles, evolving the features they needed for their prolonged flight times. Fossil specimens discovered across the world tell us that their early swift ancestors were probably small, insectivorous birds which lived in forests, so not too dissimilar to the ones that we see today. The swift fossil record is limited, as their lightweight bones are fragile and don't preserve easily, but what we do have offers an insight into their evolutionary history and the environmental factors that influenced their diversification and survival over millions of years.

Oh, I could really do with seeing the first swifts of the year now, on this mundane Monday morning, ignored by my children. I need that joy.

8.29 a.m. With the performance near enough completed, children suitably clothed, teeth brushed, and packed into the car, we are as usual, 'pushing it' timewise.

'Where is your lunch box?'

# SWIFT

My youngest child, George, looks at me like I've just asked him to solve world peace.

'I didn't see it,' he replies, despite me having pressed the oversized, bright blue lunch box packed with treats into his hands just minutes ago. The clock now says 8.31 a.m. Great, we are going to be late. To ensure we aren't, I need to be pulling out of the drive no later than 8.25 a.m., but realistically that has probably only ever happened once. I sigh and take the key out of the ignition, get out of the car and return to the house. The lunch box is on the floor in the centre of the entrance hall. Of course it is. Not even going to question it at this point.

A sound in the distance grabs my attention. It's familiar. I'm sure it's just my mind playing tricks on me. Wishful thinking on this Groundhog Day morning. I try to ignore it as I lock the lunch box safely away in the car boot, but the noise is edging closer, getting louder, and I begin to hope. Yet the chances of me reading Lev's post this morning and actually seeing a swift are so slim, I reckon it's just another bird making a funny noise. Or the neighbourhood starlings playing tricks on me. My bird call game is still not my strongest point, but still, the swift screech is pretty distinctive. It can't be, can it?

'MUMMY, SWIFT!' Jack screams from the car's passenger seat.

He's looking through the sunroof, eyes wide, brimming with excitement. He often announces birds that aren't there. A vulture in a Yorkshire woodland, an albatross in Sheringham while we ate our chips, but his energy at the moment is too real to pass off as the work of a young child's imagination.

## THE LIFE-AFFIRMING MAGIC OF BIRDS

I cast my eyes towards the red tiles of the roof, where he's looking, and squint against the patch of sun bursting through the dusty coloured cloud. And there it is.

A single swift glides effortlessly across my eyeline. I have waited since last summer to see a swift again and emotion swamps me. I think it's the fact that I know how much this single bird has fought to be here with us, although it's unaware of my existence, I'm sure. The miles it has covered to return here are an attempt secure a future for its species. It's covered twenty-five airspaces, thousands of miles and treacherous conditions, all to be here. It puts it in perspective: here's me, juggling work contracts, moving house, commuting to London and the demands of being a parent. All of that seemingly unimportant in comparison to the work that this tiny bird, which weighs less than a couple of AA batteries, puts in just to survive. And here we are, together.

The excitement of this miracle supersedes the knowledge that we are late for school. My children and I talk about the journey the swift has just been on; we wonder if it's one of the same birds that nested here last year and imagine what it must be like to fly non-stop for most of your life. Pulling up in the school car park, we realise the time and run through the gate and into the office.

'Sorry we're a couple of minutes late,' I say to the receptionist before she admonishes us. 'We spotted the first swift of the year above our house!' I am met with a blank look as she asks me to sign the children in.

As I bid them goodbye and leave the school grounds, I can't help but be filled with a mixture of delight at the unexpected turn of events this morning, and the anxiety at the same time thinking about the future of this Red List species.

The UK Red List for birds is, as it suggests, an assessment of 245 commonly occurring bird species into a traffic light system to denote their conservation concern, red being the most at risk of national extinction. Green indicates a species of least concern, Amber, those in decline. The latest version of this report, published in 2021, placed 70 species on the Red List, and 103 and 72 on the Amber and Green Lists, respectively. Most concerningly, one-quarter of the UK's birds are now in the red category, more than ever before. Joining swifts on the list are nightingales and cuckoos, both with iconic songs that we cannot possibly lose from our landscapes. Swifts fight so hard to be here with us, but what are we doing to fight for them? It was a surprise to me to discover that swifts were in so much danger here. How can that be? A bird which fights against the odds to travel millions of miles in their lifetime, and which I've watched glide with such ease in the sky above me. A species that has evolved to survive so meticulously over millions of years: how can they find themselves on a list of critically endangered species? The answer, of course, lies with us humans.

Swifts never used to be an 'urban species'. And that's mainly because 'urban' is only a relatively new concept (in the grand scheme of the Earth's history, I mean). They would have naturally nested inside caves and in trees. I have an image of a palaeolithic landscape, millennia before humans began settling in one place and curating the environment to suit their own needs, one in which swifts, in their natural surroundings, rode the air, free. Not anymore.

The Caledonian forest of Scotland plays host to the last remaining population of tree-nesting common swifts.

As humans have encroached on the natural world – it always feels weird separating humans from it as we are, of course, all intrinsically linked – we have replaced trees with concrete and removed those areas where swifts would have nested once upon a time. Swifts, like many other species which can be found in urban areas, have moved with the times and adapted to the new environment, nesting in inaccessible spaces like cracks in walls and underneath roof tiles. Swifts return to the same nesting sites every year with their life partner, but as old buildings are knocked down and renovated, replaced with new-build housing estates that don't have the same structural cavities necessary for a successful swift nest, they suddenly find themselves without a place to call their summer holiday home. Combine that with dwindling insect numbers and you have a recipe for a rapidly declining population.

The BTO (British Trust for Ornithology) and RSPB (Royal Society for the Protection of Birds) estimate populations of British swifts have fallen by around 60 per cent in twenty-five years and that number is expected to continue to fall. But, okay, enough doom and gloom, we are here to focus on the positive, after all, and there are some pretty amazing people dedicating their time and energy to the survival of the swift.

Picture this scene. It's November 2022. You're at Speakers' Corner in Hyde Park. You spot a woman who is all but naked, her body painted in intricate feathers. She is speaking about a bird, a bird which is in danger. But there's a simple solution that could mean the difference between life and death for this species and she is asking the government to act. She marches through the streets of London to Downing Street where she reads out a letter to current prime minister, Rishi Sunak. In her letter to him, she says, 'Please acknowledge our walls also belong to adventurers.'

Meet Hannah Bourne-Taylor, an author and campaigner. She can only be described as a whirlwind, a tornado, a force of nature and the driving force of the UK's Swift Brick Campaign. Born out of a passion for wildlife and a desire to make a difference, Hannah's campaign has gained international recognition for her bold, theatrical approach to addressing the decline of swift populations and other Red List cavity nesting species in urban environments, and her determination for change. Inspired by similar successful initiatives in other countries, Hannah decided to focus her efforts on trying to secure cavity nesting habitat in new builds through the national scale installation of 'swift bricks'. Simple and inexpensive, swift bricks provide artificial nesting habitat in buildings that otherwise have zero nesting opportunity for birds reliant on them to nest and breed. Given there are four Red List cavity nesting birds – swifts, house martins, house sparrows and starlings – and united in their plight thanks to loss of existing nesting habitat, swift bricks are not just a simple solution, they are also deemed urgently essential by ornithologists and conservationists for the recovery and stabilisation of these rapidly declining species. Despite this simple solution, there are no legal requirements to incorporate swift bricks into designs, and only a handful of local planning authorities have incorporated swift bricks into their planning conditions.

Swift bricks are made from environmentally friendly materials such as recycled plastic and wood, and mimic the natural nesting sites that swifts prefer, providing them with safe and secure places to breed and raise their young. By installing these bricks in buildings, Hannah hopes to create a network of nesting sites that will help to support and sustain swift populations for generations to come. It really is a simple solution. The Netherlands already have legislation in place which protects nesting sites year round and ensures swift bricks are incorporated into new builds. If sites need to be blocked for whatever reason, they mitigate by installing swift bricks or nest boxes. Easy, right? Unfortunately, the former government under Rishi Sunak declined to act and at the time of writing, the new UK government, still dragging its heels, has yet to make a decision.

I wanted to know Hannah's reason for dedicating her life to this campaign. Her response was simple. '*The birds are my why.*' Specifically, her incorruptible loyalty to birds but especially swifts.

In Hannah's book, *Fledgling*, she describes her experience of raising and releasing a swift in need of help; it was then that she fell head over heels in love with the species. When Hannah saw that the swifts' habitat was being lost at an unprecedented national rate, she realised that without these simple bricks, there would be no guaranteed habitat in the UK. New-build developments prevent the nooks and crannies that swifts need to nest, meaning that with a sharp increase of such developments popping up, there is a national-scale loss of cavity nesting spaces. The former government's budget for renovation and insulation was one billion pounds, and was set to increase to over £6.6 billion by 2023. While this is a valuable and in some case life-altering affair for humans, it means that we are blocking existing nesting sites which swifts are site loyal to, and possible nesting sites for prospecting birds.

Hannah, like many of us, believed that as an ordinary nature lover with no political power or expertise, she could just enjoy nature and someone else more experienced and qualified would solve the problem. She quickly realised, however, that no one was coming. The stats were out there for all to see, and yet there was no movement. All that data and no one was acting on it. The thought of swifts becoming extinct in the UK was unbearable.

'The idea of the last swift in Britain looking at me and asking me why I didn't do anything was not something I could live with.' So Hannah made up her mind to do something about it and two years on, at the time of writing, although she hasn't achieved what she set out to, every day she wakes up and knows she must carry on. The reality of being an 'accidental campaigner' has derailed Hannah's whole life, yet luckily for swifts she is committed and tenacious. Swift bricks are, in reality, a small and simple biodiversity measure, but they have the power to be life saving for this species. Cavity nesting birds are our closest neighbours, nesting in walls and roofs that we have built. For an apparent nation of nature lovers, the idea of not protecting a bird which shares our homes, that is a long-standing member of communities, seems outrageous. Hannah tells me she could do with a holiday, but much like swifts which spend life on the wing, there is no time to rest.

Hannah tells me that the petition method is the best option for the UK public to engage with the government. As with most things, there are good points and bad points to this system. All a petition does, assuming it gets enough signatures, is commit the government to raising the topic in Parliament; it is under no obligation to act. Yet this is still important as it lets the government know that there is wide public concern about this issue, and it raises awareness of a cause to political champions. It never occurred to Hannah, nor me for that matter, that there are politicians who want a reason to get behind a cause and that it makes it much easier for them if it's a public concern. And, surely if enough people care, then they have to listen, right? *Right?*

Hannah concludes that petitions are an empowering tool to get the public to move for a cause they are passionate about. '"Lobbying" is just a political term for "hustling". And more people need to hustle for what they are passionate about.'

I asked Hannah, what's next? 'I have no idea, I haven't achieved anything yet so I'm still focused on this,' she responds. While I can understand where Hannah is coming from when she says this, I have to say, I wholeheartedly disagree.

Hannah, if you happen to read this, you have bared your soul physically and emotionally for the species that you have dedicated your life to. You have got a nation talking. You have been the voice for these birds in Parliament when no one else would listen. You got swifts on the radar of so many people who, like me a few years ago, had probably never even noticed them. If your actions make one person put up a nesting space for swifts, and that person encourages another person to do the same, then that snowball effect will have been because of you. So, keep fighting, you glorious force of nature.

I've been lucky enough to meet several people like Hannah, who inspire and lead by example. I had the pleasure of sharing a conversation with another of these people, Chet Cuñago. It was an emotional conversation that made me realise just how powerful we can be when we make the decision to act for the causes we are passionate about. Chet lives in the Peak District and spent years walking in the rolling moors that surround her local area. It wasn't until she reached her mid-forties that birds crept into her life. A brown bird on a beach caught her attention and she Googled exactly that: *brown bird on the beach* – a story all too familiar to me. The results showed her that this was a turnstone and that began a journey of discovery and curiosity. Chet told me that she couldn't believe that she'd walked on the moors for years without spotting a lapwing, their multicoloured plumage standing out against the Peak District's often bleak landscape, or, at least, once you notice it. Chet is part of a women and non-binary birding group and describes her birding experience as 'absolute joy'. But discovering birds isn't where Chet's story ends. Rather, it's where her story begins. An awe-inspiring tale of passion and dedication.

When Chet was quite early on in her birding journey, she saw that the Derbyshire Wildlife Trust were hosting a 'Swift Party', an event designed to get people interested and invested in the species. It was taking place at a very normal, 1960s'-era house that happened to have thirty-five swifts nesting in the roof space. Drawn in with the promise of Pimms and cake, Chet arrived and saw as many as fifty swifts in a 'screaming party' above the house.

'Fifty screaming swifts above me, I'd never really noticed them before, but it seemed that for them, flying was like breathing, effortless. It felt like they had lost their connection with the Earth, ethereal beings that were more elemental like the wind, than animal.'

Chet went on to tell me about a man named Charles Cough, who started a group called All Things Swift when he realised there were injured swifts being found around the country during the short breeding season, but there were no databases connecting people with the very few specialist swift rehabilitators. He created the Swift Taxi Service, and that is how Chet first became involved in the rescue of swifts. Chet and the other swift taxi drivers would spend time looking through local Facebook community groups to find what turned out to be a surprising amount of people who were reporting finding 'strange birds', and not sure what to do with them. I can imagine finding a swift, unable to move comfortably on the ground, part bird, part bat. It would be an unusual sight!

With a limited number of swift rehabilitators at the time, Chet found herself having to look after the birds that were being found, learning from others how to care for them and the special methods needed to feed them. One particular year, Chet recalls, people stopped phoning ahead and just brought swifts to her door during the peak of a heatwave. The baby birds, unable to regulate their temperature, would move themselves to the edges of the nests in an attempt to find cooling air and would fall out. The birds in Chet's care were unable to lower their body temperatures by themselves and were at risk of dying. Fans in the house were not working, and the only thing she could think of was to enlist the help of her neighbours on the street. Every person scrambled to help, turning on their car engines and running the air conditioning, so that the swifts could be placed in the cold air. It brought to mind a memory I have of my mum dealing with a Staffordshire Bull Terrier with heatstroke when they owned a boarding kennel, rallying around to bring comfort to the distressed dog. At this point in our conversation, I had tears in my eyes and expressed my amazement at the community spirit of her neighbours, every one of them acting selflessly to help these alien birds.

Chet tells me that she didn't lose a single bird that year. An incredible testament to her determination – and that of the people around her – to protect the species which means so much to her. During lockdown, Chet gave swift boxes to her neighbours, adding ten new nesting sites to the local area.

'Swifts are like aliens when they are in the sky, spending their lives on the wing, but when they are in the rescue care, they become just like any other vulnerable bird, needing round the clock care to give them the best chance to pull through.' Chet continues, 'The four-month breeding season feels a bit like a self-imposed prison sentence, but I wouldn't change it. Once they are ready for release, their wings unfurl and they become swifts, joining the elements where they belong.'

If you ever think that you, just one person, can't have a momentous impact, think of people like Chet. Now I want you to pay attention to another incredible thing that Chet pulled off. She received a message in 2022 to say that the local council in Sheffield was undertaking a project to repair 5,000 roofs in the area. This meant that scaffolding was blocking the entrance to multiple swift nesting sites and the swifts, returning for the summer breeding season, would have nowhere to raise their chicks. After some frantic calls to the council, the work was halted. Today, Chet along with a team of volunteers, assist the council by surveying houses to ensure reroofing projects don't impact on swift breeding season. Chet used her voice and her passion and managed to have a profound impact on the future of swifts in her region. That's a lot of young swifts which would have been missing from the UK skies that year if she hadn't leapt into action. So, next time you think your actions won't make a difference, think about Chet, how one woman can make such a powerful difference to so many individuals and a bird species' survival. Remember, we have the power to change a world. Perhaps not *the* world, but someone's world. Our actions have consequences so we may as well try and make them positive and meaningful.

At the time of writing, the swifts are here with me. Screeching outside my house, sailing over the garden as they swoop for insects to feed to their chicks. For the next three months, we will no doubt announce every single swift sighting. You know when you're driving and you announce cows or sheep to whoever else is in the car with you? Don't lie, we all do it. It's like that. Just for birds. It means I stop walking in the middle of the road in my local town when I hear them overhead as the dusk parties come to life, swooping and screeching between the rooftops, while it seems no one else notices. Occasionally, I wonder how people can go about their business and not turn their eyes skywards at the sound and the aerobatic display. But then I remember how I spent most of my life totally unaware of the existence of swifts, as though I wasn't tuned into the right frequency. Once I found them, however, they became intertwined in my life and one of the highlights of our summers – mine and my children's.

Over the last few years, I have found myself noticing swifts in unexpected places – soaring over the top of St Paul's Cathedral, swirling around Big Ben, and even diving through the centre of Manchester. I hear them in TV programmes, often used incorrectly in the middle of a wintry scene.

'Mummy, all these people haven't even noticed them,' George, my youngest, announced as we watched a screaming party above the middle of our local town. We, it seemed, were the fortunate ones.

If I'm being quite honest, like really honest, after a month or so, as more swifts arrive over the garden, the sound begins to grate on me. (I know, I'm such a hypocrite.) The unmistakable screeching rubs against my eardrums, hitting all the wrong places, as we sit in the garden in the evenings. Then, a swift dives down as low as the hedges and we lock eyes for a split second, or an outstretched wing brushes past my nose as I'm putting the bins out. I'm transported on an epic journey of discovery, danger and survival, and I realise how lucky I am to be in the same place as these birds. I realise that we need to fight for them, to ensure we, my children, their children, continue to have precious moments like this.

Whatever time of year you happen to be reading this, keep the story of the swift with you, and as summer approaches, get ready to change how you see and hear the environment around you. Once you begin to notice things, there's no going back. Gaze in awe at the species which, for millions of years, has been living on the wind, travelling to the moon and back, ethereal, elemental. And try to remember the stories of people like Hannah and Chet. People who are so passionate about something that they are willing to change their whole lives in order to impact on their world. So, while you may not be able to change the entire world by yourself, there's a strong possibility you can change *a* world.

Soon, the swifts will be going, beginning their journey back across Europe and on to Africa, crossing through twenty-five airspaces and taking their song with them to share with people across oceans, thousands of miles away. The sky will be empty here, as though someone has taken an eraser to a starry night. There will be silence. An orchestra without a conductor.

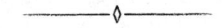

———◊———

It's August and I open my phone to Twitter. I'm greeted by another post by fellow swift lover Lev Parikian:
*I think the swifts have gone.*

# 3
# STARLING

*'I'll hollo "Mortimer,"'*
*Nay, I'll have a starling shall be taught to speak*
*Nothing but "Mortimer,"'*
        – Henry IV Part 1, Act 1, Scene 3

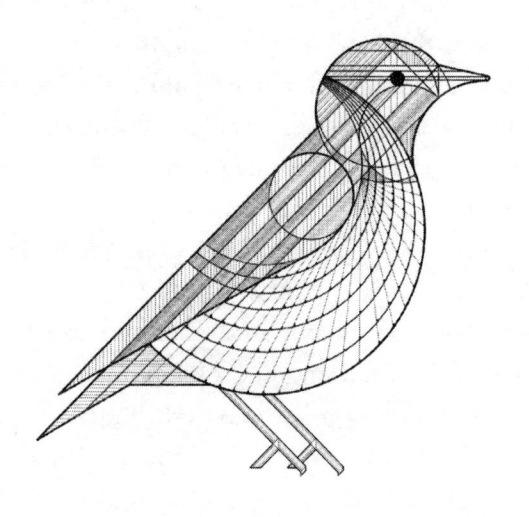

**Look for the unexpected**

It's December 2023. A high-pitched squeaking noise stands out against the hustle and bustle of Borough Market and grabs my attention for a second. I'm leaning against a wooden post, a box of chips in my hand from one of the many food outlets that surround me. Hundreds of people mill around: couples holding hands, families with prams edging their way through the crowd. From my perch at the side of the raised seating area, I have a perfect view of the entire space and spend some time watching the tourists taking photos and locals rushing through, rolling their eyes impatiently when someone unknowingly blocks their path. It's my first time here and, having lived in a rural part of the country for a while now, I jump at any opportunity to surround myself with crowds of people in lively cities. And the more time I spend here, the more at home I'm starting to feel in London. *There's that squeaking noise again.* It reminds me of a dunnock. I remember Nick Acheson, the king of bird sounds, once describing a dunnock sound as a bike that needs oiling as someone pedals it down the street. I look up to see the green metal structure which holds up the dirty, stained canopy above our heads, swaying gently in the wind, which is picking up. As the structure moves, the noise continues. Now I've noticed it, I'm finding it hard to focus on anything else.

A black shape opens its wings and, as I watch, its beak opens, and I hear the annoying squeaking sound perfectly replicated as the bird starts a solo performance. After a few moments, it flings itself from one of the green metal beams and hurtles towards the seating area in search of scraps. *A starling.* Looking back at the beams, as my eyes tune into the shadows, more and more starlings start to appear, much like when you're staring hard at the night sky and more stars reveal themselves.

I didn't come here today expecting to see nature apart from a pigeon or two along the river. I should have learnt my lesson by now. I find nature in the strangest of places and now I find myself looking into the eyes of a starling which has landed, confidently, on the post I'm leaning on, eyeing up the food in my hand.

# STARLING

If you've never seen a starling up close, please make it your personal mission to do so as soon as possible. You may never have noticed a starling. But once you see them and learn about them, then prepare to have your world turned upside down. Okay, let me try and paint a picture with words for you, though admittedly, no words can truly describe the gift that nature gave us in starlings. They are small birds, about the size of my hand – that probably doesn't help you I know, I could have massive hands. On first inspection, you could be forgiven for thinking they were just black, and perhaps a bit shiny. But look again and you will enter an entire universe hidden within the feathers. When the light catches a starling, the black plumage bursts into life, and like light bouncing through a stained-glass window and on to a church altar, an iridescent array of purples and greens shine back at you. Each feather along the starling's breast looks as though it has been carefully crafted, hand painted by a talented artist with a small white heart. As it takes flight, this glossy obsidian figure transforms into a metallic disco ball, casting its colours out into the world.

Starlings can be seen around the UK all year round, but they really show their true colours, so to speak, during the winter months where they take to the sky in aerial ballet displays, known as murmurations, swarming in groups of up to one million birds, filling the sky in a carpet of individuals moving together to form intricate shapes across fields, above buildings, and perhaps most spectacularly, in seaside settings where they can be seen dancing above piers against pastel backdrops as the sun sets. My favourite fact about starlings?

Males have a blue splodge at the bottom of the bill and females have pink. We don't subscribe to gender stereotypes at all, but it's fun to spend time with my kids looking for the pink lipstick to identify the female of this species!

Like all of the birds we've met so far, starlings come with their own fascinating history. The common starling, or the European starling we see in the UK, is thought to have originated in the Mediterranean before spreading to other parts of Europe and Asia; it's even found now in North America. And how they came to be in North America is fascinating in itself.

Imagine the scene.

It's 1890. A man called Eugene Schieffelin, and his staff, have just signed for an interesting and expensive delivery which they carry across New York City. They head straight for Central Park with their interesting cargo, which has never been seen in America. You see, Eugene, like myself, was a massive Shakespeare fan and he came up with a misguided plan to introduce every species mentioned in the works of Shakespeare on to American soil. This guy was persistent and, with little contemporary knowledge of ecology and the potentially damaging effects of introducing a new species, he opened a cage and sixty starlings took flight, filling the skies above Central Park in the first American murmuration. (That last bit was added for dramatic effect, and may or may not have happened like that.) The following year, he imported another forty starlings and did the same thing.

Over half of the original one hundred died, but thirty-two of them took hold in New York. In just a couple of decades, they had reached the Mississippi River, and today they can be found in every state from Alaska and as far as Mexico! Populations are soaring at over 200 million individuals, making them a commonly seen bird, although locals across the country have mixed feelings about this non-native species. For a bird that was only ever mentioned once by Shakespeare, starlings have had a huge impact on the US. I wonder what Shakespeare would feel about that? Would he be happy that his work had such a lasting effect, or would he be mortified at the way Eugene tried to honour him? If only the Bard had known then the impact he would have when he wrote that one sentence in his play *Henry IV*: 'I'll have a starling shall be taught to speak / Nothing but "Mortimer," and give it him / To keep his anger still in motion.' Shakespeare was, of course, referring to the incredible mimicking ability that starlings have.

I have a confession to make. The story about Eugene Schieffelin has been proven to be nothing more than an urban myth. Eugene became chairman of the 'American Acclimatization Society' in 1877, and their aim was to release non-native flora and fauna in North America. It's true that the negative impacts of non-native species were little understood back then. There is also evidence to suggest that Eugene's starling introductions in the 1890s were not the first time they had been released into the country and, in fact, evidence suggests the first release took places twenty years before this by another acclimatisation society in Ohio. So, while the Shakespeare story might not be true, it certainly grabbed my attention and imagination, and it's easy to see how stories like that can quickly take hold and be considered fact.

With advanced auditory processing skills and a complex syrinx (a bird's vocal organ), starlings have unmatched abilities to recreate the sounds from around them. You may find city starlings mimicking police and ambulance sirens; in Borough Market, they copy the squeaking of the metal beams that hold up the overhead canopy, or, like parrots, they can copy human voices and even schoolchildren's laughter. The starling on my roof likes to impersonate a screaming swift and has even confused me with a convincing *'peep'*, making me look around for an oystercatcher. It amazes me to think that Shakespeare and I both recognised the incredible uniqueness of this bird and, four hundred years apart, decided to write about them. I'm not comparing myself to Shakespeare's greatness, but I am suggesting that, even in the middle of bustling Elizabethan London, people stopped to notice nature.

In the UK, it's a different story. Starlings find themselves on the Red List of species at risk of extinction: we are down to just 1.8 million pairs. In Britain, we have a habit of filling in holes in buildings and removing trees that aren't 'just so'. Our obsession with tidiness has stripped the starlings of their cavity nesting spaces, and without them the population will fall. I saw a news piece recently about a neighbourhood in East Anglia where the residents were complaining about the noise and mess that was being created in their housing estate by nesting starlings, and demanding the council relocate them. I'm not sure how they planned on relocating birds. Asking them nicely to move? This level of disconnect breaks my heart. The joy I feel every time I see a glistening starling on the bird feeder in my garden is just magical. The starling which sits on the roof mimicking the noise of a swift, even after the swifts are long gone, reminds me of the brilliant interconnection between the species that I can see from my doorstep. If we continue to plough forward without change, then we will continue to lose so many natural treasures from our landscape. And what a quiet, grey, joyless place it would be without them. I remember the first time I saw a starling. No, let me rephrase that. I remember the first time I *noticed* a starling. Of course I'd seen them before, but I hadn't *seen* them. So, let's rewind again to September 2021.

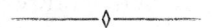

---

Liverpool is, and always has been, special to me. Despite never having lived there, it's one of two places on this big planet that feel like going home. With a dad in the military, we moved around a lot during my childhood, and I never had the opportunity to live near family or put down roots in a place. Despite living literally on the opposite side of the country, I try to make the trip back to Liverpool as often as I can to see my family and, most importantly, my grandma.

My grandma is an important character in my life. She was one of the stable pillars during my childhood, moving around so much. When we lived in Hong Kong, she was there. When we moved to Yorkshire, she was there. To France, guess what? Yep, she was there. It's only now that she has landed back in Liverpool, and I'm on the other side of the country, that we have been apart for long periods. I feel guilty about that. I feel bad that we don't make the trip more often, leaving my mum to do the running back and forth to visit her and take her to appointments, but life just seems to get in the way. My grandma and my mum are the two women who got me to where I am now. It sounds clichéd as hell, but without their support I don't know where I'd be. I hope they know. Perhaps

I should tell them how grateful I am? Perhaps we should all let the ones we love know how much we love them?

Each time we visit Liverpool, we usually end up in Kirkby to pick up some essentials. Now, Kirkby is an area of Merseyside, around six miles from Liverpool, that is characterised by its market and small town centre. Rows of covered stalls, selling everything from Marks and Spencer's kids' pyjamas to fruit and veg, feature in the market, opened in 1960, and draw people in to wander around to see what bargains can be claimed. Kirkby has a long history; in fact, it's been known as a settlement since AD 870, when Alfred and Aethelwold were fighting battles against the Danes. It's hard to imagine that when you're wandering around B&M. Kirkby makes an appearance in the Doomsday Book under the name Cherchebi, meaning 'church village'. In the 1950s, Kirkby was selected as one of the areas to be made into 'new towns': large housing estates to support the overspill from surrounding cities. And now, it's often a busy little town with families exploring the charity shops and my grandma getting her cream cakes from the Pound Bakery, which does exactly what the name suggests.

We abandon the car in the large flat car park and wander slowly across the main road towards the town centre, with one thing in mind before we look inside any shops – chips and a coffee. Jack and George run ahead of my mum, grandma and I, stopping at the thirty-foot, silver statue of an elephant on a boat. I look at the elephant which is holding a spear in its trunk and greet it with the same befuddlement that I always do. Every time I see this statue it seems more and more bizarre. A Google search does me no favours either. An elephant on a boat? I've got nothing. As far as I know, there aren't any records of elephants frequenting the market in search of some knock-off Nikes.

There's a tiny café at the entrance of the market. It's scruffy, usually full of pigeons, cheap and, most importantly, really, really friendly. Something that I miss when I visit my own local shops is that characteristic friendliness of Scousers; they really are brilliantly unique.

'You okay, what can I get you?' A small woman speaks to me from behind the counter. Her black fleece is hidden by an apron she is wearing over the top to protect from the greasy food that is spitting at her from where she stands.

There's nothing like a decent greasy spoon. Sitting back at the table and emptying ketchup sachets and packets of sugar out of my pocket, my grandma has always used one too many sugar packets in her tea. 'Do you want some tea with that sugar?' I'd say. 'It's only a teaspoon's worth,' she would reply. A bloody big teaspoon.

The kids scramble for their drinks, and a couple of chips fly through the air in the mad dash to grab their food. My own seagulls, only here for the chips. George wobbles the table and my mum's tea splashes over the side of the cup. 'George!' Mum exclaims in mock sternness. I smile at an older man who is sitting on his own at the table next to us and has looked over the top of his paper to watch the commotion. 'Left me bird to do the shopping while I put me feet up, maybe you should do the same,' he announces cheerily in quite possibly the strongest but warmest accent I've ever heard. He picks up his copy of the *Liverpool Echo*, where I can see Jurgen Klopp staring at me from the back page, and takes a sip of tea from his mug.

## THE LIFE-AFFIRMING MAGIC OF BIRDS

A woman appears at his side, short white hair in tight curls and a lilac coat that comes down to her knees, buttoned down as far as it will go. She pops a Pound Bakery bag on the table, and smiles at us. 'Soft lad trying to chat you up, is he?' She laughs, poking her husband affectionately.

'He was telling us about his bird,' George, my chatty, confident child, pipes up through a mouth full of chips, not realising the man was not talking about the feathered kind.

Yet, the woman dives into her carrier bag and, to my surprise, pulls out a small bag of bird food which she opens and offers the boys. 'Here y'are, do you wanna give this to the dicky-bird?'

My heart warms when I hear her say that. 'Dicky-bird', a phrase rooted in Cockney rhyming slang which seems to have made its way up north and reminds me of my grandma when I was a child, feeding the dicky-birds, usually robins now I think about it.

The boys scramble about. The bird doesn't move; in fact, another two have joined it in the hunt for crumbs. As they sprinkle bird food on the floor, I look back at the café staff, who seem nonplussed at the scene.

'They're funny little birds,' the woman continues, sitting down next to her husband, 'they make all kinds of noises, don't they, Jim?'

'Sounds like car alarms sometimes at home or sirens. Make me get out of me chair to check out the window to see if the bizzies are coming,' Jim says, rolling his eyes.

'Well, something needs to get you out of the bloody chair or you'll grow roots,' she responds.

We didn't exchange any more information about the birds. We didn't discuss their name or marvel over their unique

# STARLING

appearance or their mesmerising winter displays. At the time, I didn't know about this unique behaviour, I didn't even know what the bird was. But what we did was come together to have a conversation. For a moment, a couple of birds on the lookout for some food brought us together in a moment that has stayed with me. Nature has the power to do that. It has the power to bring people together. It has the potential to introduce you to new things, new people, new friends and new experiences. It's incredible how something that is literally just there, in front of you, can go unnoticed for so long. I'd never noticed a starling before. But once I did, I knew I needed more and I began to seek out those new experiences that nature had proved to be able to offer me, unaware of whom or what nature would eventually lead me to.

I know I said the staff didn't seem bothered about us feeding the starlings that time, but returning to the café recently, I spotted a large 'Don't feed the birds' sign outside the neighbouring food outlet, Martin's Deli, home of the famous Kirkby sausage. It seems that Martin isn't as much of a fan of the starlings as Jim and I.

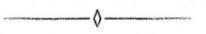

---◊---

'Are you staying for the murmuration?' a warden in a bright blue jumper asks me. It's February 2023 and I'm walking towards the visitor centre and car park with every intention of leaving RSPB Minsmere for the day and heading to the car for the two-hour drive home.

Pretending I know exactly what a murmuration is (I've never seen one so I'm guessing), I say, 'I guess I could.'

'You should,' the warden replies excitedly. 'It's a huge murmuration. There are about twenty thousand birds that come in to use the reeds to roost. They spend their day in smaller flocks and then all come in from different directions to join up in one massive flock. It's really amazing. You should stay, if you can.'

Turning around to face the direction I just came from, I trek back through the reserve until I reach a stretch of path flanked by reed beds on either side. Presumably, judging by the fifty or so people facing in the same direction, that's where I need to be looking. As I follow the direction of the fellow onlookers, I am greeted by a massive power station that stands out against the landscape. There's no blurring of lines between nature and humans here; our impact on the environment is plainly obvious, and it's in the shape of Sizewell nuclear power plant. Now that I've seen the backdrop, I'm less excited to see a natural spectacle unfurl before me. How can any natural spectacle look impressive with a great big dome that reminds me of the Death Star in the middle of it?

As we stand and wait, the temperature dropping, I scan the scrub in front of us. A muntjac deer wanders across my field of vision, seemingly unaware of the audience. I'm starting to shuffle around as boredom and the cold creep in through my thick hiking coat. A child next to me sits down by my feet and begins picking stones out of the path, leaving holes where they once were. He throws a couple of stones at my leg before his mother pulls him away, apologising, but I laugh and reassure her there are worse things in the world than having some gravel thrown at my leg.

'Look, they're coming!' another child shouts excitedly. This one is slightly older and stands behind his granddad's scope, which is pointing upward towards the power station.

## STARLING

As I move my gaze away from the now holey path, I see a group of birds in the distance rise up from the ground, quickly followed by more and more black shapes. There is a snowball effect as more birds join the group, and as they travel upwards, they are now a massive, rolling ball, moving as one across the sky. The sun is setting, painting the sky with pastel shades of pinks and blues, reminding me of a Bob Ross painting tutorial. As though someone has dipped a paintbrush into a selection of watercolours at once and dragged it across the sky, 'a happy little accident'. The white power plant starts to blend into the background, blurred by a haze of light cloud covering it. The aerial procession of birds pulls our attention away from the intrusive building as they dance their choreographed routine and form intricate shapes as they move like synchronised swimmers going for Olympic Gold. Suddenly I realise that the human impact on the land does not take away from the spectacle that is happening in front of me – in fact, if anything, it shows me how adaptable nature is. It teaches me that no matter what, nature will prevail, perhaps in a different form, but to quote Dr Ian Malcom, 'life finds a way'.

———◊———

It's November 2023. I've seen a lot of incredible images and videos of urban starling murmurations with them tumbling across the skies of coastal towns. The one that stands out in my mind is a huge flock swirling against a stormy sky over Brighton pier. I haven't had time to go to Brighton as the autumn draws to an end, and so I decide to head to the next best thing available to me, Great Yarmouth, where there is apparently a daily murmuration in the town centre. Now,

## THE LIFE-AFFIRMING MAGIC OF BIRDS

I've heard mixed reviews about Yarmouth, but I'm keeping an open mind in the hope that it's going to prove to be an awe-inspiring place filled with incredible and heartwarming moments in nature – you never know.

I pull up in a car park with the kids after doing loops of the town centre, my sat nav failing to direct us to the seafront, only to discover that this car park is so far away from the water that we may as well be in Brighton. We trek through the town, stopping so the kids can sift through baskets of seaside tat in shops that look as though they are undoubtedly a front for another kind of business, and eventually see the calming sight of the still sea, framed by a perfect blue sky.

'RIDE,' my youngest son loudly exclaims as he spots the snail merry-go-round, and a ghost train tucked awkwardly behind a sign that reads 'Joyland'. Brightly coloured snails with suspicious expressions painted on their faces stare at us, and I imagine them slowly taking underwhelmed children round and round in circles. Unfortunately, Joyland appears to be closed today so we are just going to have to discover our joy elsewhere. I breathe a sigh of relief until I realise we are about to walk along a whole street dedicated to amusements. The bright colours scream from the buildings at me; Peppa Pig shouts 'Hello' from a dilapidated ride sitting next to a machine designed to electrocute those who decide to stick a pound in and have a go. Hundreds of dodgy looking Pikachus capture my children's attention from grabber machines, and I do my best to usher them past with the promise of a fiver on the 2p machines later. They protest as we walk towards the quieter end of the beach which stretches out in a clean sheet of gold sand.

## STARLING

I hear a familiar robotic series of sounds calling from above and look up into the currently disused Ferris wheel. It reminds me of a film I saw once about the abandoned fairground in Chernobyl. There's nothing quite like the British seaside. The starlings are sitting above us, sheltering from the wind which is now picking up as we get closer to the water. As we watch, more and more appear like stars in the night sky once again. I stand and watch the starlings for a while as the kids cover themselves in sand. In a few minutes, they will both run up to me moaning they have sand in their eyes and demanding we never go to the beach again. How long are we supposed to wait for a murmuration? Do they perform a show every night? Is it a guaranteed spectacle? All these questions run through my head as I wonder if the ninety-minute drive was worth it.

'Mummy, George threw sand in my eyes. I *hate* the beach,' my eldest child screams as he runs towards me, his younger brother following behind with a mischievous grin on his face.

'I threw sand at Jack's face,' he declares with absolutely no regret in his voice. He rattles as he passes me, pockets full of stones that I will find at a later date stored in various crevices in the car. I only hope he hasn't slipped a crab's leg into my open handbag. Again.

Giving up, we wander back to the amusements, and I unwillingly hand over a five pound note for them to change into 2ps and gamble away as they try to win a single Drumstick lolly that's been sitting in the machine since 2014, or a tiny squishy toy with googly eyes that will undoubtedly burst all over one of them at a moment when I don't have any wipes or a sink to hand.

## THE LIFE-AFFIRMING MAGIC OF BIRDS

As the sun starts to get ready to set, I usher them out of the amusements so as not to have to navigate across Great Yarmouth town centre in the dark to get back to the car. I'm disappointed not to have seen a murmuration. I seem to keep missing them, but then again, their performance is not for me alone, and I can't demand a private showing just because I happen to be here. Peppa Pig shouts 'Hello' again and I look to see what kind of ride the voice is coming from this time. As I do so, my eyes widen and I fling my arms out, startling the kids as I tell them to 'Stop!'

Silently grabbing both of their hands, I pull them down the side street towards a small church which is hiding quietly behind the chaos of the seafront. They protest and question what I'm doing until they realise that above the church are thousands of individual figures gliding effortlessly against the wind that whistles around our cold ears. This is the closest I've ever been to a starling murmuration. As I stand directly under them, they create a 'whooshing' sound as they breeze past. Tiny patters like raindrops hit the ground around me as they pass their droppings mid-flight, some hitting my coat, but I don't care. I can feel myself grinning as I witness this spectacle. This unexpected, magical show. This performance feels like it's just for us.

I turn around as I hear voices and see a couple of other families standing and looking up at the sky. All of us sharing in this moment. I notice two women in their pyjamas, sitting on the wall outside their house with cigarettes hanging out of their mouths, pause their heated argument to watch as the starlings take a lap of honour past them. A man in a dirty green coat steps out of the corner shop, two bottles of vodka clinking in the white plastic carrier bag in his hand.

## STARLING

He stops as though someone has pushed him backwards as he notices the scene in front of him, and he smiles before weaving his way down the road away from us. Humans, from all walks of life, coming together as one, pausing for a moment, taking ourselves away from whatever is going on in our lives and sharing this privilege together. At this moment, we all just happened to be in the right place at the right time. This show would have happened whether we were here or not, but today – for one day – we all got to experience it. Together.

---

February 2024 and it's one of those late winter evenings where the season is really taking hold and making itself known. I remember The Holt Bookshop, my local bookshop, posting on Instagram about a nearby starling murmuration and, as I drive home from the school run with my kids in the car, I decide to pull over to see if they responded to my message asking where it was spotted. I'd love to see a murmuration so close to home but I'm not feeling hopeful. I pull into a parking space on the way into the town, switch off the engine and load my messages on my phone, stopping only to turn up the heating as the temperature starts to drop.

'Look, Mummy,' the voice of my youngest son calls from the back seat of the car, 'murmuration'. I half acknowledge him, knowing that he calls every flock of birds he sees a 'murmuration'. (I'm still not entirely sure when a group of birds moving together becomes a murmuration; it's a bit like trying to work out when a pond becomes a lake.) I assume it's the local feral pigeons doing their hourly lap over the tops of the houses.

'No,' my eldest son knocks on the window to draw my attention upwards, 'there actually is.' And sure enough, when I look up, I gasp as a thick, black blanket flies directly over the car.

Gazing up through the sunroof, I can see hundreds of individual bodies making up the sheet of birds that tumble through the sky, expanding and contracting like a diaphragm taking deep, purposeful breaths. The cloud of starlings turns back on itself and moves towards the fields, and as we watch them vanish slowly into the distance, my kids chatter excitedly about how cool that was to witness. As they settle back down, my youngest burying his head back in his book, I start the car and move in the direction of home.

These unexpected experiences are what fill me with the most joy. Turning my head upwards to see a whole world moving around you in a place where you didn't expect it to be is what keeps me so engrossed in nature. The ever changing, ever evolving way that nature greets you each time you step out of the door is what fuels my desire to open my eyes and find the unexpected in every moment.

Do me a favour, when you put this book down – step outside your front door and just look around you. On your walk to work, look up at the branches of the trees. Stop as your kids examine the leaves on a hedge outside school. Pause and look around you, notice nature, find the unexpected. Let those unexpected moments fill you with childlike wonder and take that with you every day as you battle through the stresses of life. Nature is, and always will be there. Whether you have already connected with it or not. It's there, so you might as well have a look.

# 4
# PEREGRINE

*'Friends, Romans, countrymen, lend me your ears . . .'*
*— Julius Caesar*, Act 3, Scene 2

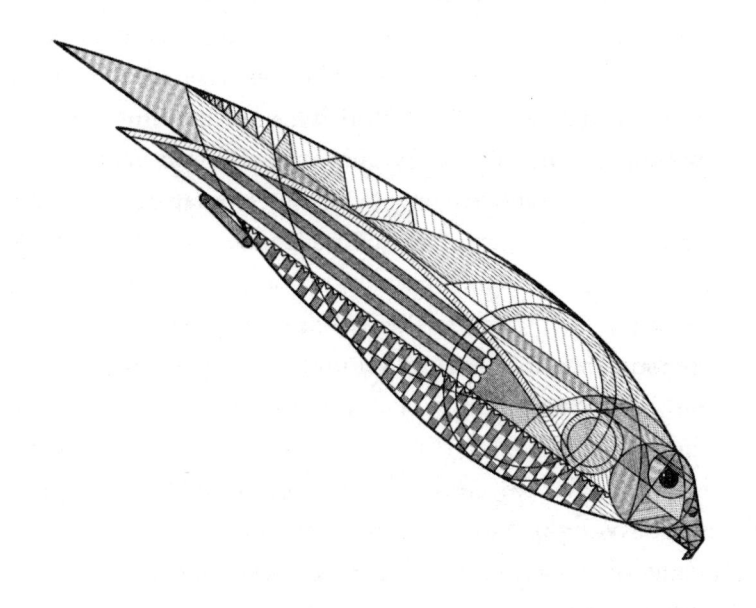

**Learn from those who are there to teach**

'PEREGRINE!' Jack, my eldest, exclaims, as a bird flies past us on the Norfolk Coastal Path.

As I look at the bird in question, the dark shape disappears over the only hill in Norfolk and into the distance, leaving only a distorted image imprinted on my imagination. I will admit my bird of prey ID skills are still significantly lacking. To me, peregrine, sparrowhawk, merlins, hobbies, all look like pigeons in flight. I can just about tell the difference between a red kite and a buzzard – if I see them from the right angle. Otherwise, they're all just big birds that I will be distracted by happily as they circle over the car when we are on road trips.

It's 2023 and Jack has never seen a peregrine in real life before. He's admired them on videos and photos for a while, though, and I don't want to dash his dream if it was, as I suspect, a pigeon. We continued to walk, Jack excitedly chattering about seeing his first peregrine, me keeping quiet. As we turn a corner, he slams his arm into my stomach, stopping me in my tracks, and before I can exclaim, he points to a bird perched on a fence-post. I whip out my phone camera and zoom in, the binoculars in the car. And he's right: it *is* a peregrine. We stay in the moment for a while, before we head back to the Wildlife Trust visitor centre to grab a drink and buy yet another book that I don't need from their excellently stocked book section. Old habits and all that.

As we climb the stairs, a tall, white-haired man stands, leaning casually against the banister, grasping the enormous lens which hangs around his neck. Jack stops and, in a rare and unexpected and odd moment of excitement, as he normally avoids talking to strangers at all costs, announces to the man that he has just seen a peregrine.

My delight at his sharing his joy at this experience in nature quickly fades and I want to shrivel up into a ball as the man replies dismissively, 'So? I've seen hundreds. It's only a peregrine.' I expect Jack to be disheartened by this negative encounter, but overhearing this exchange, a kind volunteer steps in and shares in his delight. 'Woah, that's cool! Fastest bird in the world, aren't they?' He's looking at me as I mouth 'thank you', my son's wonder at seeing the peregrine untouched.

Let's pause for a second. I'm not for a second expecting every person on Earth to stop and indulge my sons. I'm aware that not everyone wants to speak to children, and some people don't wish to speak to anyone at all. But this mean-spiritedness towards a young child who was simply trying to share his delight at the magic that had just unfolded in front of his eyes is not the first and I'm sure won't be the last such encounter. I'm not asking everyone to share in the excitement if they don't want to. But it's not a competition. We were all at the beginning of our journey at some point. We all have experienced that childlike wonder when, as kids, we saw a butterfly float in front of us, jumped in a muddy puddle with our wellies on, delighted at the sight of a duck eating bread at the local pond. We have all had these incredible moments and it's important to remember that. It's a bit like driving (and this is an odd analogy, so bear with me because it's how I see it).

Picture the scene. You're coming up to a roundabout, stuck behind a learner driver. The learner, L plate waving in your face, slows to 15 miles per hour as you approach the roundabout and stops when the road ahead is completely clear. You get frustrated. You gesture and unnecessarily mutter, 'you could have got ten tractors round there by now'. The learner eventually pulls off and they feel the absolute thrill that they just made it round a roundabout for the very first time. They're celebrating inside. You, on the other hand, enter the roundabout feeling disgruntled, forgetting that once you were that learner driver, feeling that sense of elation and success. Wherever you are in your journey with nature, whether you're a child who has just seen a peregrine for the first time or a lifelong birder who has travelled the world seeing thousands of species, we've all had that feeling of utter magic, so let's allow each other to enjoy the moment, and take that with us as we explore the world together. Be it in on your own backyard or in the jungles of South America, the magic is there waiting for us. It's a choice, so choose kindness: you'll feel better.

Peregrine falcons are pretty cool, so my son was right to be excited. Possibly one of the more iconic and fascinating birds of prey in the world, they are known for their immense speed and agility. Female peregrines are the larger of the species, though, unless they were next to each other in a line-up, I'm not sure I'd be able to tell the difference in the sexes. In a dive, known as a 'stoop', which is how they catch their prey, they become the fastest thing in the animal kingdom, reaching speeds of around 200 miles per hour as they hurtle towards their prey. To put this into context, the fastest land animal, the cheetah, hits speeds of about 61 miles per hour in a sprint. Peregrines are like avian torpedoes, literally and metaphorically. They have a structure inside their nostril called a tubercle which helps to slow the air, minimising the force; otherwise they might be prone to passing out mid-flight. Their strong flight muscles and pointed wings, lined with stiff feathers, make them the perfect shape to bomb through the sky, stopping only when they collide with their prey, usually an unsuspecting pigeon. A live-action demonstration of Newton's first law of motion.

As a history fan, I feel compelled to give you another bird origin story, and the history of peregrine falcons is long and has intertwined with human civilisation for thousands of years.

They captured the imaginations of artists and in religious symbolism going as far back as the ancient Egyptians, whose god Horus was depicted with the body of a human and the head of, you guessed it, a peregrine falcon. Horus symbolised power and divine authority, which if you think about their incredible, effortless speeds, isn't far from the truth and you can see how that came about. Perhaps the most well-known appearance of peregrines in history is during the medieval period, when they were often used in falconry, trained to hunt small game. Those of you who have ventured into Middle Earth may remember that hobbit Pippin's full name was actually 'Peregrine Took'. Who knows, perhaps Tolkein had been wowed by the aerial force of the bird and was so inclined to name one of his most notable characters in honour of them. Amazingly, the peregrine is found on every continent except Antarctica, from Arctic tundra to rainforests, and in urban areas they've adapted to nesting on tall buildings as a proxy for their natural cliffside nests and, perhaps most notably in the UK, on cathedral spires.

Now, I want to cast my mind back to the first time I noticed a peregrine, or rather, the first time a peregrine was pointed out to me in a moment that I only recently realised was one of those key times that set me on the course I find myself on today.

---

It's April 2019, I'm nearly a year into an archaeology degree at the University of York, unaware that next year the world as we know it will be flipped on its head when a global pandemic will rage and shut everything down for a while. For now, I'm ignorantly wandering through the city centre on the way to collect my children from nursery. I haven't spotted my oystercatcher yet, I haven't had that magical moment of reconnection with nature, that joy is yet to hit me but it's coming soon, whether I know it or not. My kids' nursery is situated in a beautiful part of the city, tucked right under the Minster and sheltered by a canopy of trees that create shadows on the Yorkshire stone paving slabs underfoot.

I usually walk straight across the front of the Minster, the towering medieval construction looming over me, my eyes pulled not towards to pigeons and the jackdaws at my feet who are waiting for the crumbs of the many tourists enjoying their lunch on the stone steps, but to the incredible stained-glass windows which run along each face of the building, adorning the structure in bright, colourful pages, each one telling a different story. Easily the most notable of them is the Great East Window, an early fifteenth-century work of art and the largest example of medieval stained glass in the country. It's said to depict the beginning and the end of everything and, once you see it, it's easy to believe it so. It's impossible to paint a picture of the window without seeing it. Even photos don't do it justice. To give it some perspective, it's about the size of a tennis court. If you stand in front of it at just the right time, when the sun is setting, the low light shines through and illuminates the entire piece, each ray highlighting an individual story from within.

Today, I feel the call of the window, tempting me to go and spend yet more time marvelling on the art, recently restored in one of the world's most complex historical conservation projects, and costing a cool £11 million. But for some reason, I stray from my usual path. I'm a bit early and have time to explore before getting the boys, so I take a quick detour and head for the Minster gardens instead. Walking through the black iron gates, I am greeted by groups of mums, with prams, sitting on the grass on picnic blankets while their barefoot babies crawl and toddle about around them, couples enjoying ice creams despite it not quite being 'ice cream weather' yet, and a runner being pulled by a large husky which is attached to a lead round her waist.

A man is sitting on a bench in front of me as I round the path towards the Chapter House.

He's wearing a brown jacket and is sitting with one leg crossed over the other, his arm casually draped over the back of the bench. He is staring up at the top of the Minster where the stone gargoyles meet the grey lead roof. As I draw closer, I get the strange feeling that I recognise this man from somewhere, but I can't quite place him. Thankfully, he hasn't noticed me looking at him and, as I am about to walk past him, it hits me where I know him from.

'Mr Hickenbottom?!' I stop in front of him.

He starts, pulling his eyes from the Minster to look at me. 'Hello?!'

'Charlie Bingham, you taught me physics, like, fourteen years ago,' I offer, as I'm sure he doesn't have a clue who I am. I wasn't exactly a natural in his physics classes.

'Yes, of course, I recognise you, what are you doing here?'

'An archaeology degree, late bloomer, mature student on paper.' I use my fingers to create quotation marks around the words 'mature student', trying to lighten this unexpected encounter. 'Amazing place to sit and take in the sights, isn't it?'

Mr Hickenbottom – Francis as I now know him, which still feels weird despite being a thirty-two year old with my own children – points up at the roof of the Minster.

'Peregrines. If you look for long enough, you'll see them. They nest up there and hunt the pigeons.' And there's the same subtle excitement in his voice I remember from the days when he tried desperately to teach me second-year physics and I just as desperately resisted.

Remember, at this point, nature is not on my radar. I have an idea of what a peregrine is. I wouldn't know it if I saw one sitting on the roof of the Minster. In fact, from a distance I would probably assume it was a pigeon.

I didn't realise this encounter would stick with me, that later it would make me look up at every cathedral on the off chance that something awesome might be perched at the top. I'm still in touch with Francis. In school, I never realised he was such a massive nature nerd, and perhaps if I had paid more attention as a teenager, then I could have learnt a lot from him. Instead, I'm making up for it by intently following all of his Facebook posts on the weird fungi and bugs he spots during his retirement. If I could give a piece of unsolicited advice at this point it would be this: if you have a teacher who is passionate about something, listen to them. Learn from them. Embrace their passion and share in their joy. Who knows, they may just alter the course of your life, much like my unexpected encounter with my physics teacher has done. And Francis, if you're reading this, thank you for sharing that moment with me. You may have forgotten it, an insignificant moment in your life, but for me it was the beginning of a turning point. I just didn't know it yet.

---

So now that my experience of historical cathedrals has been permanently altered, it's April 2023 and I find myself sitting under Norwich Cathedral with my children and a promise of some peregrines. I'm quickly realising that just rocking up with no actual knowledge probably, in this instance, wasn't the smartest move. Especially after promising a child a peregrine sighting. If you don't know, Norwich Cathedral is massive and, like York Minster, is old. Nine hundred and twenty-eight years old, in fact. Well, that's when it was started at least, when William II had claimed his seat at the helm of England.

Perhaps my favourite part of the cathedral is the bosses that decorate the ceiling and detail the Creation story with bright colours and intricate artwork. Over 1,000 of them, in fact, the largest collection of medieval bosses in any cathedral. Bosses are the finely decorated underside of keystones which are essential to the construction of cathedrals. They are often intricately carved and sometimes, as is the case of Norwich, painted into individual works of art which together tell a story.

The collection of 'Green Men', more commonly associated with paganism, stands out too, with their gold leaf making them glisten as the light plunges its way through the stained-glass windows. But today we are not here to marvel at the architectural genius of medieval stonemasons; we are here instead to attempt to marvel at the nature which calls the cathedral home. We do a couple of laps outside looking up at the building and keeping our eyes on the sky. It's a fruitless exercise. We leave, disheartened by the lack of peregrines, lifted only by the promise of a Pizza Express on the way back to the car.

Luckily it doesn't take long for us to make up for the distinct lack of peregrines that day. Fast forward a couple of weeks,

## THE LIFE-AFFIRMING MAGIC OF BIRDS

I've dragged the kids into Cromer on a hunt for some new school shoes. There isn't a huge selection of shops in the town so I'm not feeling hopeful about the excursion, but with the children growing like weeds, it seems necessary. Suddenly we share the same shoe size. The main part of Cromer is just one long street with gifts and charity shops lining both sides and an Iceland taking centre stage opposite a medieval church.

But Cromer is a fascinating place with history weaved into its core. It was a small village in the eighteenth century, but the Georgian obsession of heading to the sea to cure all manner of ailments and complaints, led to the gentry expanding the town and building a lot of the beautiful buildings still seen today. The local rich families sent their relatives to the town as it was easier to travel to than the popular resort of Brighton, and having now lived by the sea for several years, I can see the logic behind that. There's nothing quite like a bit of sea air to 'blow away the cobwebs', and there's sometimes nothing more soothing than just seeing the choppy grey waves and smelling that 'seaside smell', which I believe is actually the scent of bacteria devouring dead phytoplankton and pheromones produced by seaweed. Yum. The narrow streets of Cromer that lead to the sea were once used as smuggling routes and are said to be haunted by the ghosts of travelling monks. A book on Cromer's history by Walter Rye, published in 1889, tells tales of a gruesome, blood-covered spectre that wanders the churchyard.

It's now in that very churchyard that I find myself. Instead of gruesome ghouls, however, we have unexpectedly found ourselves among a group of people with scopes pointing towards the church spire. I get chatting to one who tells me that they are part of the Cromer Peregrine Project and, during nesting season, they often pop up in town with their scopes to engage the public and show people what's living on their church spire. Shoppers and tourists wander past without so much as a sideways glance, but I watch as the volunteers actively encourage passers-by to come and have a look and learn about the nature on their doorstep. I peer up at the top of the church and can see a tiny dot looking down at the town, surveying the area. Looks like a pigeon to me.

'Peregrine', Jack, my eldest, shouts.

I turn around and see that one of the volunteers has lowered his scope to allow him to get a glimpse of his favourite bird. He stands captivated, looking through the scope for a few minutes before his brother pushes him out of the way to look for himself. Not wanting to miss out on the action, I wait until George retracts himself from the scope and bend down to reach the level of the eyepiece. I stand at the base of the old church, squinting, trying to keep my left eye closed as I look through the magnifying lens. I've always struggled to look through scopes and binoculars. For some reason, scopes give me an instant headache and binoculars make me feel like I've got motion sickness.

High above me, the peregrine falcon perches, its sleek body perfectly poised, unaware of the spectators marvelling at him. The sea breeze is strong today, whipping around the old stone of the spire and ruffling the feathers. Each feather moves in a delicate dance, catching the light and shimmering. I watch, captivated, as the falcon seems to scan the horizon, its sharp eyes ever vigilant. The wind carries that seaside smell as a scent of chips wafts through from the nearby chippy. It's a sensory symphony, the sounds of waves crashing in the distance blending with the chattering of tourists exploring the high street and the cars at a standstill trying to get through the narrow, one-way street. The bird remains unperturbed, an effortless king of the landscape, every movement precise and deliberate. The peregrine shifts slightly, adjusting its stance. Its feathers ruffle and settle, a display of effortless grace. I feel a sense of awe and privilege, witnessing this moment of wild beauty. It seems strange to be standing in the middle of a busy town watching this seemingly mythical beast. A bird that I've always assumed was inaccessible to me and now I can spot it nearly every time I pop to Iceland for the weekly shop! The falcon seems almost otherworldly, a creature of legend perched on the spire that has stood with the peregrines through centuries of change. *Magic.*

We take the coastal route back to the car, walking along the clifftop with the sea to our right. Black-headed gulls linger ominously, floating as though suspended by an invisible wire, riding the wind as they eye up the sandwich in my hand. They're waiting for the perfect opportunity to swoop in and have a taste. I throw up a tiny piece of bread and a gull expertly tackles another mid-air in order to catch the treat. A figure whooshes past at head height, zooming along the clifftop in the opposite direction, back towards town and the church. A family behind us are too busy arguing about what to have for tea to notice, chippy or cooking in the caravan? I know which I'd choose, and I reckon the gulls would agree.

'Peregrine', Jack says again.

It strikes me that I have been to Cromer several times a week for the last few years and yet I'd never seen the peregrines. Or have I seen them and just not noticed, just not really looked? How many other species are around me? How many insects beneath my feet, birds on the nearby beach, undiscovered wonders? That's why nature is so magical to me.

A late diagnosis of ADHD came at a time when I was rediscovering myself after children and after completing a degree with great difficulty, not understanding exactly how my brain worked (add in a global pandemic for good measure and I'm not entirely sure how I graduated). As a child I was constantly met with school reports that contained phrases like, 'has potential if she would only apply herself' or 'lacks commitment'. Turns out, I just wasn't being channelled in the right way. Nature was the first thing that, once I rediscovered it, I never let it go. It transpired that the ever changing, constantly evolving nature of nature meant that my newfound obsession wasn't just another craft or hobby I could master and then move on from. It wasn't an instrument that I could work to pass the highest-grade exam and then switch to another.

Every time I leave the front door and step out into the open, I see something new. Whether it's a peregrine at the top of a church I've walked past for the last two years and failed to see before, or an oystercatcher wading along the shore, nature is constantly moving and, by that definition, you can never get bored of it! So, as this book is meant to be about the lessons nature can teach you, I want to give you a challenge. When you next go outside, or when you look out of the window, or stand on your balcony, put your phone down (unless of course you're using it to take photos or use an app to ID your find), and find one new thing. I swear to you, unless you're underground in a sterile nuclear bunker, nature will be in front of you and you will spot something, maybe several somethings, new. It may be a pigeon on a roof or a bit of weird moss on a brick wall, a funny looking leaf on a bush or a worm the like of which you've never seen before on the path, but it will be there.

Go outside, notice nature. Repeat.

Keep doing that until there's nothing left to find. Warning: once you start, you'll never be able to stop. Admittedly, there are *worse* addictions.

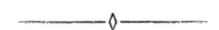

---

It's March 2024 and my phone's just pinged with a text from Chris Stone, a Norfolk birder who is always on hand to send me information on anything interesting that passes through. 'Eagle in Glandford', it reads.

It was Chris who first told me about a death's-head hawkmoth (think the *Silence of the Lambs* movie poster, you know the one with the moth covering Jodie Foster's mouth). Never in a million years did I think I would be rushing to a local beach to ogle a moth, but times change. What do all those memes say, one day you're young and hip, the next you're setting a birdfeeder cam up in the front garden. Guilty as charged.

We've been here before, sometimes not that successfully. Chris has texted before and I've driven half an hour down the road, only to be told the bird in question has just disappeared off into the distance and doesn't look like it's coming back. So, I'm not hopeful about the eagle, but as it's just a few minutes from the house and we are just about to go in that direction anyway, we may as well have a look.

Pulling up at the location, there are a couple of people set into the hedges with their scopes, looking at something, and yet still I don't feel hopeful. I tuck my car out of the way and bundle the kids out. Of course, my scope is in the living room as I've been using the tripod for that garden birdfeeder cam, and my binoculars are in the suitcase that sits unpacked from our recent holiday. Eagles are pretty big, though, so I'm counting on the fact that I'll be able to see it. Right?

We walk along the road, dodging cars which honk at the 'twitchers' and gesture unkindness towards them despite everyone being stood safely out of the way. Stopping at a man whose name I unfortunately didn't ask, we stand next to him and George, the youngest, who isn't normally overly bothered about birds, unless it's a St James's Park parakeet that has landed on his arm, suddenly shouts: 'There. It's like a brown triangle next to the wonky tree.'

Sure enough, sitting calmly on a branch in the distance, next to a fallen tree, a large brown triangle surveys the landscape. The man standing next to us, upon witnessing the excitement of the kids, immediately beams and adjusts his scope so that they can get a proper look at this, our first eagle. I'm not going to pretend to know why there's an eagle sitting in a tree in Norfolk when they don't live here, and to be honest, I don't really have much of an interest in finding out right now. All I know is that at that moment we had the most amazing opportunity right on our doorstep, and we were lucky enough to share in that experience with others who were there for the exact same reason.

Our kind neighbour shares that he doesn't really know much about the birds either, but he does experience a huge amount of joy from these experiences. He tells me that while some get pleasure from exotic species on foreign shores, he gets as much pleasure watching the sparrows in his garden at home. For him, what matters is the beauty of it all and making sure it's still there for the future generations to enjoy. And what better way to ensure the future generations care than to immerse them in it, captivating them and allowing them to keep hold of that wonder. I see that in my boys.

As we continue chatting, my youngest looking through the scope and exclaiming at every movement and ruffle of the feathers, I scan the immediate vicinity for my eldest son, who has disappeared from eye level. He has taken root on the wet, grassy floor below our feet. Not wanting to seem rude and interrupt the conversation, I wait until a natural break in our chatter and dip down to join him in the mud. He sits on his knees, leaning forward at an awkward angle with his hands behind his back. I don't mimic his position; my core strength (or lack of) would have me tumbling forward face first into said mud.

'What are you looking at?' I ask him, curiously.

'That.' He points at a disturbingly large pink squiggle that is concertinaing its way across the ground. Before I can reply, he continues, 'Good isn't it? It's so weird, and long and pink like a pig. You can't drown a worm.'

I wonder how or where he learnt this fact. But it is sort of true that worms absorb oxygen through their skin, so they can survive being submerged in water as they simply sip up the oxygen from the water around them. A useful skill to have with the UK climate. I smile, standing up before my knees seize up.

I look around me. The adults are all staring at the spot where the eagle can still be seen. Then I glance back at Jack, who is still on the ground transfixed by the worm. It strikes me that the eagle is certainly spectacular, a huge spectacle, naturally drawing crowds. I mean, come on, it's an *eagle*. Unless I get in the car and drive for twelve hours to the north of Scotland, or head to the south coast of England, my chances of seeing one are fairly slim, so I'm not knocking this experience. But, isn't that worm just as spectacular? A species that is quite literally vital for our life here on Earth, and yet one that goes unnoticed and, in some cases, it's something that people are averse to.

Let's pause the bird talk for a second and imagine a world devoid of earthworms, which spend their lives eating and recycling organic matter to keep our soil healthy and 'clean'. Without them, the intricate balance of ecosystems and, of course, our agricultural practices would suffer huge alterations, reshaping the very foundation of life as we know it. Sounds dramatic but it's true. Soil structure, once enriched by the tireless burrowing of earthworms, would gradually become compacted and impenetrable. The absence of these delightful decomposers would disrupt the cycle of nutrient recycling, leading to depleted soil fertility and diminished plant productivity, so farmers would struggle to grow enough crops to keep our growing populations fed. Without the tunnels created by earthworms, water regulation in soil would falter, rendering landscapes more vulnerable to flooding and runoff during heavy rainfall. The repercussions would ripple through our ecosystems, including our beloved birds, as earthworms, a vital food source for many organisms, vanish from the food chain. Ultimately, the disappearance of earthworms would echo across the fabric of existence, underscoring the intricate interdependence of all living organisms within the complex tapestry of nature. To put it plainly, a world without worms would be pretty rubbish. So, if you think about it, the tiny worm, wiggling its way through the damp grass, is worthy of as much awe and wonder as the white-tailed eagle which is passing through. The worm is a stark reminder that nature literally is all around us, even if we can't see it. The worm tells us of an unseen story that is happening beneath our feet even when we aren't looking. A world full of creatures which most likely don't realise how important they are to the giants above them, just like a lot of those giants don't realise how much we depend on them. Next time you see a worm, try not to recoil in horror. Try and see it for what it actually is. A remarkable engineer. An artist, unknowingly sculpting our society with its creation. And thus concludes my love letter to a worm.

In that moment, the unsuspecting worm taught me a lesson. No matter how small I feel, how insignificant I may feel my actions are, they're having an impact somewhere. So if you're feeling uninspired or like your efforts at work or home are fruitless, or like what you do doesn't make a difference, remember the worm.

You're important.

You're vital.

You are enough.

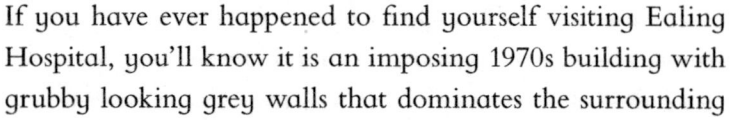

---

If you have ever happened to find yourself visiting Ealing Hospital, you'll know it is an imposing 1970s building with grubby looking grey walls that dominates the surrounding landscape. I unexpectedly find myself looking at this landmark in the distance as I stand in the shadows of Wharncliffe Viaduct, a Grade I-listed structure, built by Isambard Kingdom Brunel in 1836, as part of the Great Western Railway. It's April 2024 and I'm with Dr Sean McCormack, a vet and the founder of Ealing Wildlife Group. He's pointing up to a huge stone crest that lies flush against the brickwork.

'Freddie usually sits on the unicorn when he's not incubating eggs. See what he's left behind on the unicorn's head?' He's chuckling at what could be mistaken for white paint splashed down the head and body of the poor unicorn.

Freddie and Dusty are the Ealing peregrines. Sean admits to influencing the decision to name them after two gay icons, Freddie Mercury, lead singer of Queen, who attended Ealing Art College, and Dusty Springfield, whose real name was Mary O'Brien, Irish singer who used to live in Ealing. Other suggestions were Rachel and Carson, the first and last names of the 1960s pioneering environmentalist who, in a proper act of girl power, wrote a book called *Silent Spring* where she took on the agricultural industry to fight against pesticides. Her book predicted what would happen if we continued to use the contemporary pesticides, and how bird populations globally were suffering as a result of DDT, a revolutionary pesticide which was being used to kill off pests and produce amazing crop yields. DDT had a huge impact on birds of prey, particularly peregrines and sparrowhawks which eat pigeons. As grain eaters, pigeons were consuming the laced crops, which would then accumulate in the peregrines. It didn't make them infertile, but their eggshells became so thin that they were breaking on the nest before they had the chance to hatch. Numbers crashed globally and they were faced with extinction. Rachel Carson's movement saw these pesticides banned, and eventually the affected bird of prey species began to recover. Sean told me that some fifteen years ago when he first came to London, there were around twenty breeding pairs of peregrine in London. Now, they're bouncing back fantastically with an estimated fifty pairs now in Greater London. 'Look up on any tall building in London and chances are you'll find a peregrine,' he tells me. 'I'm rubbish with bird of prey ID. I don't think I'd know if a peregrine flew over me in the city,' I admit, ashamed that still I can't tell my peregrines from my sparrowhawks. 'Ah, it's all about the jizz,' he replies, chuckling at my reaction.

Let's address the elephant in the room. Jizz, for those who don't know, is, in this case at least, a phrase that stems from the term, which was used in the Second World War for identifying military aircraft and stands for *General Impression of Size and Shape*. It's a term that's been used in birding since around 1921 and refers to the identification or exclusion of a combination of characteristics to confirm or deny a species identity. Yeah, I'm not really sure what that means either. Basically, to give you an example of something I don't fully understand, you see a friend on the street, and based on a number of known characteristics and features that you know to be true, you can identify that person as your friend. Jizzing, in birding, is exactly the same. You utilise the characteristics you know about a species to deduce its identity. I'm still not sure that's going to help me with my bird of prey ID, Sean. Sorry.

Sean shows me his phone screen where he has connected to the peregrine live camera which is currently looking at Dusty, a female incubating her eggs, high up on an specially crafted platform installed on the hospital by Ealing Wildlife Group. Sean tells me to be on the lookout as Freddie, her partner, isn't on the nest so is likely to be having a break nearby. After a final sweep of the viaduct to see if Freddie is lurking above our heads, we carry on walking in the direction of the hospital. The noise from the busy road crescendos as we approach, and I look down at the long grass we are walking through that has been left unmowed. Yellow dandelions peek out from between blades of green grass, bringing the sunshine down to the ground for us. A dandelion never fails to cheer me up. So many people seem to think of dandelions as needless weeds. But how can the fuzzy balls of brightness fail to bring a smile to anyone's face? If anyone asked what my favourite flower is, I'd actually be inclined to say a dandelion. The name 'dandelion' is said to come from the French, *'dent de lion'* meaning 'lion's teeth'. I'm not sure I understand the name 'lion's teeth' – perhaps *'boule de soleil'* would be more appropriate? They're vital sources of food for those all-important pollinator species like bees, and they absorb nitrates from the soil. They're resilient and will usually spring back no matter how much you chop them down. There's another lesson to be learnt from that, I reckon. In this world which can often seem pretty gloomy, I don't think anything negative can come from leaving the balls of sunshine to thrive. What is life without a bit of colour, after all?

    I bend down while Sean continues to look at the peregrine camera on his phone for signs of Freddie and pluck one of the dandelions from the ground that has transformed to its white fluffy puffball stage. It transports me back to my own childhood, walking across the sprawling wild lawn in front of Nostell Priory, an eighteenth-century Palladian manor in West Yorkshire. Barefoot and holding hands with my mum as we travelled across a blooming meadow of dandelions and stopping to wobble the seeds out of the puffball flowers.

I think of my favourite photo of my son George. He's two, his wild long blonde hair curling around his ears. He's holding a dandelion up to his face, eyes closed in silence, cheeks puffed out ready to release air through his slightly parted lips to send the seeds and his wish swirling through the light breeze.

I gently blow the dandelion that is hanging in my hand and the individual seeds parachute into the air, beginning the next stage of their journey. Maybe I'll come back next year and see another happy dandelion that has planted itself from my brief interference. Music has always had the power to evoke strong emotions, but I never realised before that moment that flowers have the power to transport me back to memories from my past, and for a brief second, I smile and I'm six again, holding my mum's small, warm hand as we dance through the dandelions.

After another five minutes, chatting as we walk, we are standing by the busy road and the sounds of the aggressive London drivers beeping their horns at stationary cars, cyclists whizzing past, impatient engines revving overwhelm me momentarily. Then I remember why we are here. Standing in Ealing Hospital car park, I look up to where the peregrine nest is and spy an avian outline perching on a windowsill round the corner of the building, feathers blowing slowly in the breeze.

'There he is.' Sean points to where Freddie is taking a break from incubating eggs and delivering food to his partner.

# PEREGRINE

In the wild, peregrines would naturally nest on cliffs, but of course, as we encroach on their spaces, like many other species, they have to adapt and find suitable urban nesting sites. The box that was installed by Sean as a collaborative project between Ealing Wildlife Group and Ealing Council is not a bird box like you might imagine. It's more like a wooden cat litter tray of gravel which acts as a substrate to hold the eggs in place and prevent them from rolling around. Pigeons are a favourite food source of the peregrine, and here in London they are abundant. Sean tells me that, when watching the cameras recently, he saw two brave (or stupid) pigeons land directly on the tray, like Uber Eats for the peregrine, or DeliverCoo. But they were lucky and she would not leave her eggs, even to catch such an easy snack.

There are ten species of birds of prey in Ealing: peregrine, kestrel, hobby, sparrowhark, merlin, red kite, buzzard, barn own, tawny owl and little owl. Remarkable really for a bustling borough of London. It's hard to believe that now as I stand in the grey, drizzly car park of the hospital, listening to the hum of the road and the symphony of roadworks taking place just a few metres away from me. It feels impossible that in the midst of all this chaos, somewhere in the trees behind me, or on top of the tall buildings which surround me on all sides, there are incredible species, lurking unseen.

I wonder if all the people inside Ealing Hospital right now are aware that just outside the room where someone may be recovering from surgery, or a consultant may be taking her lunch break inside her office, are two parents working tirelessly to incubate eggs and provide themselves with the energy to do so. Very soon, those chicks will hatch; then the real work will begin!

## THE LIFE-AFFIRMING MAGIC OF BIRDS

In July 2019, the Mayor of London signed a charter to make the capital the first National Park City. That in itself is a bit of a paradox. How can London, a concrete jungle with a population of over eight million people, be considered a national park? How can it compare with the other UK national parks: Snowdonia, the Lake District, Loch Lomond, the Norfolk Broads? How can London, with its towering glass buildings and overpriced housing, possibly be placed in the same category as these other areas of outstanding natural beauty?

Well, it may surprise you (it surprised me) to discover that London is around 50 per cent green and blue space, made up of gardens, canals, ponds, parks and pockets of wildlife hidden around the city. In fact, I was even more surprised to find out that London is actually considered to be one of the world's largest urban forests with over eight million trees. Imagine that, a tree for every person who lives in London.

After spending a lot of time in the rural countryside and now a lot of time in big cities like London, I've discovered that when you look for it, urban wildlife is, right there, all around you. When you open your eyes to it, it becomes impossible to miss. Whether it's a pigeon in Trafalgar Square (not anymore, the council sent peregrines in to clear them up, so the iconic Trafalgar pigeons are no more) or a fox in the middle of Hyde Park, nature is just there. And actually – and you might gasp at this – if you gave me a choice between spending time at a nature reserve in the middle of nowhere or a park in the middle of London, I'd choose the city every time. I can't explain what it is. There's just something about the contrast between those huge buildings that seem to stake their claim on the land as they tower above the streets, and the green spaces that lie just below them. It shouldn't work: 'nature city' is an oxymoron, two things that shouldn't come together, but somehow they just do. It shows the wonderful adaptability of the natural world; no matter how much we creep in on their world, they will keep fighting and keep thriving. There's another lesson there somewhere, I think.

———⋄———

It's May 2024 and I find myself wandering along Holkham beach with my best friend, Dan Rouse. She's my bird expert. She suffers daily terrible pictures and videos of birds from far away that I have seen and, most of the time, impressively is able to decipher them and accurately let me know what I've seen. She suffers and yet never complains because Dan knows that by imparting her knowledge, she's helping me on my journey and teaching me more and more about the natural world. She shares her knowledge with me, and I repay her with more dreadful photos.

Spring is on its way out and summer is approaching. The weather is doing that thing where it's not quite sure when spring ends and summer begins. It's warm, but we have our raincoat hoods pulled up to beat off the light drizzle that is falling across the open sandy beach. You know that rain that is barely there but gets you wet in minutes? 'Pissy rain', as my mum would call it, adding, 'if you're going to rain then at least do it properly.'

We drag ourselves, with very little grace, up the side of a particularly steep sand-dune to join Dan's partner, Sam, who is set up for a sea watch. (A sea watch, for those who aren't sure, does exactly what it says on the tin. You set up your scope, and watch the sea, seeing what drifts into view.)

Sam is standing next to another friend whom I didn't expect to see, Ptolemy, another Norfolk-based birder who is also watching the sea through a scope. For half an hour, we share in this moment. Just four people who are all, in our own way, passionate about the natural world. Some dedicated to birding, experts who spend their life working with birds, studying them and travelling far and wide to see them, and others (me) who just think birds are cool.

I look over my shoulder and see a bird in the distance and, nudging Dan, point and say, 'Look, pigeon,' with a grin. We have a running joke about my love for the most typically unloved bird species. In fact, I believe my photo in her phone contacts is a pigeon.

She looks, sighs, and in her strong Welsh accent, with a hint of exasperation, she says simply, 'That's a peregrine'.

# 5
# SWALLOW

*'True hope is swift, and flies with swallow's wings.'*
*Richard III*, Act 5, Scene 2

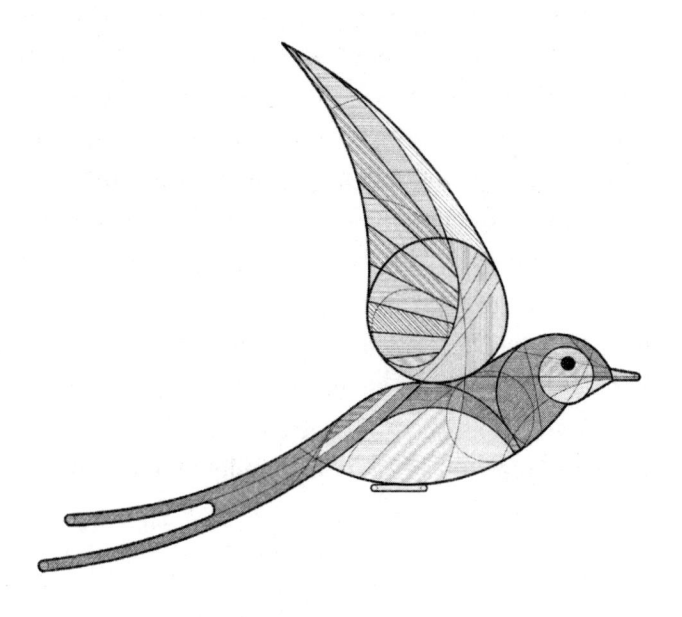

**We aren't removed from nature,
we don't own nature, we are nature**

There's a nest above the entrance to my children's school. Tucked into the eaves of the old Victorian schoolhouse, the uneven surface, camouflaged against the grey flint walls, could easily be missed by an unsuspecting eye. I imagine the bobbly mud structure could be mistaken for a wasp's nest and thus avoided at all costs by passers-by, as though a glance in the wrong direction might trigger a swarm.

This nest belongs to a small visitor, currently clinging on to the edge of the structure, head bobbing in and out of an opening. It could be mistaken for a swallow, I suppose, and not so long ago I probably would have assumed it was. Now, I can see that this bird, a member of the same family as the swallow, has slightly different features.

House martins lack the streaming tail feathers that swallows carry behind them. I always think house martins look a bit chunkier than their cousins – the swallows' less sleek friends, understated, but that's why I love them. You can sometimes spot house martins near puddles where they collect mud to build their intricate nest structures, like tiny sustainable housing developments. I'd never heard of a house martin before. And yet now, here I am, back in the playground where the other parents are gathering after dropping their kids off on the penultimate day of the summer term, looking up at the bird, again.

On first inspection she has simple black feathers along her back. But if you wait for the light to hit at the right angle, you would be dazzled by the blue tones that flash like lightning striking through a midnight sky. Her white rump shows as she twists her body trying to keep hold of her temporary home and nursery for her children. No one has paid them a blind bit of notice, except me.

'What have you found this time?' A familiar, friendly voice over my shoulder says, pulling me back to the ground like a fledgling tumbling from the nest. It's Hope, one of my 'Mum friends' who has well and truly accepted me for my quirks. 'Bird Woman', she affectionately calls me, a nickname I happily embrace. I am what I am, right?

I am now torn. Do I give her the full 'Bird Woman' response, diving into the fascinating migration habits of the house martin? Do I tell her they are hirundines, in the same family as the iconic swallows who are also tumbling through the skies in the village? Do I plead to her compassionate heart and tell her they are a Red List species, the population of which is plummeting across our skies? Should I tell her that we used to believe that house martins and swallows hibernated at the bottom of ponds, and we somehow are still learning about their movements? Does she want to know about these incredible natural pest controllers? After all, the air would be swarming with tiny insects if it wasn't for that bird sitting a few metres above me, feeding her chicks. Will she zone out as I gleam with excitement, talking about this bird that we have the privilege to share the same airspace with? Or do I give her the short answer she really wants? The mother takes off over our heads, her deeply forked tail spread out as she jerkily flies out on another hunt. The avian equivalent of me popping to the local Budgens to get something for the kids' tea, and then going back again later when I realise I forgot the stuff for tomorrow's packed lunch. Happens more often than I'd like to admit.

'It's a house martin,' I reply.

'Oh. I thought that was a wasp's nest.'

With the kids safely deposited, I get back in the car and pootle down the road for a few miles, slowing only to roll my eyes as a tractor pulls out ahead of me. I arrive at the popular birders' meeting point, the Norfolk Wildlife Trust's Cley Marshes car park. A quick stop in the empty visitor centre to show my membership card and collect a bright orange sticker to say I could enter the reserve suggests it's going to be a quiet day on the marshes, despite the perfectly clear blue sky that seems to be suspended over the calm sea. I attach the sticker awkwardly to the front of my jumper, the way a kid who had just been to the dentist would.

An overwhelmingly loud sound from a tiny Cetti's warbler startles me as I skim the hedgerow that hides the car park from the main road with my hand. Cetti's warblers are very small brown birds with skinny feet that cling to slim branches. I suppose they look a bit wren-ish to my untrained eye. The RSPB website describes them as 'nondescript' which I don't think is fair. Alright, they're another LBJ (little brown job) but they make up for that with an unmistakable call that sounds like they are shouting, *'I'm a Cetti's warbler'* (honestly, go and find a video of the call so you can see what I mean), which they bellow from the reeds and blackthorn bushes that line the path. Just as I start to think to myself, *I always hear Cetti's but never see them*, a small chestnut ball darts out from within the branches, still singing the unmistakable song, *'I'm a Cetti's warbler'*, and crosses my path.

I shove my bulky car keys in my backpack and start the day's adventure. It's July, which means the summer season is well underway, and the species I can see and hear as I walk deeper into the reserve definitely make this fact known. It feels as though they are all in the summer spirit and celebrating with joyous hoots and calls.

A soft *chugg-chugg-chugging* starts behind the line of tall trees to my left, gradually increasing like an old-fashioned steam train coming into view. I half expect the driver to sound the whistle as it passes. Only one problem there, the famous North Norfolk steam line is a few miles to the south. Or is it the west? Cardinal points never were my strength.

## SWALLOW

As the mechanical whirring edges closer, I look up to the tree line and see a large white body fly over my head. Outstretched wings and a long, thin neck tell me this must be a mute swan, the iconic bird of royal parks and humble duck-ponds up and down the country. But I have never heard a sound like this before. It doesn't sound like a bird. It sounds like a piece of advanced technology in flight.

I pull out my phone to ask Google why mute swans make such a racket when flying? I am met with several search results that basically say, 'we don't know'. The closest thing to an answer is from a website that looks less than trustworthy, which states that the sound, which can be heard up to a mile away, *might* be a way for swans to communicate with each other. I think they just like to make their presence known. Like an extrovert arriving at a party. I wish I knew that feeling. I find at large events I am more like a wren, often there but hiding in the hedgerows, trying to blend in with the walls.

I continue until I get to a wooden bridge which crosses a small channel. Pausing on the bridge for a few minutes, I lean on the railing and look down the water, back towards the visitor centre. I think this is my very favourite spot in Cley. The famous East Bank, which seems to be where most birders flock, may offer spectacular views across the whole marshes and a range of ever-changing species. But this spot offers something else. It offers peace. I've rarely seen anyone else stop here for any length of time. I've politely nodded at plenty of passers-by as their feet pound over the thin planks, but few people stop. This is the perfect place for kingfishers. Plenty of low hanging branches that dangle over the water, gently skimming the surface as the breeze sways them. Ideal perches for the electric blue bullets to hunt from. But have I ever seen a kingfisher here? Of course not. I don't think they actually exist. The unicorns of the bird world.

I leave my tranquil solitude on the bridge and join the boardwalk which winds its way through the tall reeds. The wind blows gently through them, moving the fluffy tops like ruffling a shaggy dog's head. *I haven't seen a marsh harrier yet*, I think to myself. That's one thing I've noticed about Cley: you can't pass through without seeing a marsh harrier or two soaring across the landscape. Still plenty of time, though.

Arriving at the end of the boardwalk, I am greeted with a choice. Three hides stand before me. Each one a wooden house with a thick thatched roof. Each offers up a different view of the pools that lie in wait on the other side of the buildings. Each pool calling me with the promise of a different story, different species which are busy making the most of their summer destination. Tales from Africa, countries I've never had the fortune of visiting, but the birds which are waiting in the pools are ready to tell me all about them. Or so it feels. I consider my options for a second before deciding on the hide to my left. I pull open the door and am met with darkness as the closed shutters made sure no light could permeate.

Walking into a dark space with plenty of hidden corners fills me with panic. It's something I have encountered in many reserves; the old-style bird hide that is designed in such a way that sends anxiety rippling through my body as I wonder who could be lurking. 'It's just a bird hide,' you may be thinking. But to me, a woman arriving in this dark space alone, it is the stuff of nightmares.

I take the bulky bag off my back and use it to prop open the door, allowing some light to fill the room. Then, checking that the hide's definitely empty, I proceed to open just two of the shutters. The two right in the middle that provide the best view of the pool ahead of me. As I heave them open, the stiff hinges bellow loudly. It's such a contrast to the still silence that had come before, I am surprised it didn't trigger an eruption of birds, disturbed by the almost tremendous roar coming from the wooden building, the antithesis of the surroundings. Finally, I sit down on the bench, still aware that I am alone in here, but putting that thought to the back of my mind, I look out at the scene ahead of me.

As promised, an entire world stands before me. Most noticeable is the clump of black and white figures that are floating, wings tucked beside their bodies, over the far side of the pool. Black headed gulls are a familiar sight all year round on the North Norfolk coast, and with their breeding plumage fully developed, their black heads look like they're wearing little balaclavas, perfectly contrasting against the white feathers that coat the rest of their bodies. They are such a common sight for me now that I sometimes forget how wonderful they are. Amber listed, so not entirely safe from population declines, and yet here in this moment they seem at peace and free from the stresses we humans put them under.

I go to pick up my binoculars to step into their world, a world I can't see with the naked eye, but they are not next to me. I look around and check inside my bag, which is still propping open the door, and soon realise I've left them back in the car. Again. Perhaps I won't be exploring as much of the world as I hoped. I scan the pool and my eyes fall upon two spoonbills who are standing up to their knees in the water and large enough to see perfectly without equipment.

Spoonbills, as the name might suggest, have bills, shaped like spoons. This is my kind of bird naming, say what you see and make no mistake. Blackbird, chiffchaff, pink footed goose, all examples of birds with sensible names that you can't fail to understand why they are so named. A friend recently told me that a baby spoonbill is called a 'teaspoon', and to this day I'm still not sure if they were having me on or not. I very much hope it's true. Spoonbills are brilliant birds; they spend the winter on the south coast and southern Europe, and a small number return here to the North Norfolk coast to breed. But this was not always so. Spoonbills were once a common sight in the UK during the Middle Ages. There's a fifteenth-century misericord in Lavenham, Suffolk, Britain's best preserved medieval village, that clearly depicts a spoonbill. Back then, worshippers were expected to stand during long services, so they didn't fall asleep. Misericords (a miserable name, isn't it?) were small ledges attached to the pews to give people a little bit of respite, somewhere to lean. Many of these were intricately decorated by expert carpenters. The detail suggests the artist who carved it must have been familiar with the species, much like cave paintings of lions and bears suggest a familiarity with species who are no longer locally extant. After all, they couldn't exactly get on to Google and research 'bird with a spoon shaped bill', could they?

Spoonbills often found themselves on the dining tables of royal banquets, and by the 1700s they had been hunted to extinction in the UK. Then, something incredible happened in 2010. Breeding spoonbills were discovered in Holkham,

North Norfolk! Since then, successful chicks have fledged every year, and the spoonbills keep coming back.

Sitting in a hide, watching these spoonbills, I consider this conservation success story and feel privileged to be in the company of such a wonderful, historic species. In fact, all of the species wading and floating across the pool. None of them are aware of my presence. Except a greylag goose, which I can see peering over a line of grass, watching me, guarding his world and making sure I am not a threat to his empire. Which, of course, without my binoculars, I'm not.

I decide to check out another hide. The view is the same, but sometimes a slight change in perspective can create a monumental shift. I choose to pull open the door of the middle hide, the aptly named Central Hide – say what you see – and something happens that I am not expecting. I'm still early in my birding journey and don't know what species I will encounter when I visit the reserve. I'm just out for a walk to calm the thoughts racing in my head, but this hide feels different. I wasn't met with the same darkness I experienced in the last hide when I entered. A window on the left is letting the sun cascade through the open shutter, creating a warm pathway of light that leads all the way to my feet, welcoming me in.

Before I have time to take a seat on the wooden bench, something darts in front of me and out the window, quicker than I can focus my eyes to see it properly. I dash to the opening and lean out slightly to try and figure out what it could be. Why would a bird be inside the hide? As I gaze out on to the pool, past the waders and the mechanical mute swan which has landed and is now snoozing on the grass at the edge, I notice more small shapes flitting back and forth. Without my binoculars, it's impossible to get a good view, until one of the shapes bravely soars past me, back inside the building. I look up and in a moment of realisation, I see the freshly glazed, navy plumage. Two long tail feathers hang over the beam that the swallow is perching on.

Suddenly, thoughts of my first bird story come rushing back and I am fifteen again, lying on the grass looking up at the sky. I reflect for a moment on how much my life has changed since that day. I am no longer a teenager, but a mother determined to create a successful and abundant future for my children and myself. Much like the swallow sitting in front of me, who effortlessly disappears into an intricate structure, lined on the outside with perfectly plastered mud like a woven basket, that is tucked neatly into the corner where the thick beams meet the edge of the roof. For a few minutes, time stands still and we are just two mothers sharing the same goal.

Heavy footsteps approach on the boardwalk outside, accompanied by two deep voices that grow louder until the door of the hide is pulled open. The swallow, startled by this intrusion, flits out of the open window as two large, camouflage patterned camera lenses enter the doorway, closely followed by their owners, who awkwardly mumble a 'hello' in my direction before settling themselves on benches at the opposite side of the room. A marsh harrier swoops across the back of the pool and disappears as quickly as it arrived, behind the sand-dunes in the distance.

That experience with the swallow was very early in my birding journey or, should I say, my adult journey of reconnecting with the natural world. Moments like that are exactly why birding has been a way for me to not only connect with nature but connect with myself and unlock core memories and experiences that are lodged deep in my mind. The spontaneity and the ever-changing essence of nature means that a simple walk can be transformed into an exciting adventure. Curiosity peaks with every footstep. Every second is an opportunity to learn if you take it, an opportunity to experience an entire world in front of your very own eyes.

Swallows join us every spring after completing the 6,000-mile journey from South Africa. They travel 200 miles a day, risking exhaustion, starvation and dehydration, in a bid to return to the breeding grounds. They were the stars of my first bird story, a species close to my heart, drawing me back to memories of a six-year-old child leaving the Word Museum of Liverpool with my grandad, walking with my tiny hand safely placed inside his seemingly giant palm. His fingers kept a tight hold to protect me in the busy town centre. My eye level fell upon the tattoo positioned in the space between his thumb and forefinger. The swallow looked back at me, linking us forever. If you're looking for a bird to kickstart your bird journey, they're a good one to go for. Swallows can be spotted across the UK during the spring and summer. Anywhere there is a steady supply of insects, swallows are usually there, performing effortless aerial tricks, as they scoop unsuspecting insects from the sky and tend to their young.

Fast forward a year, almost to the day. I'm sitting in the very same hide. I'm not sure how many writers choose to write from within bird hides, but it seems an apt place to be writing a book about birds. It's the middle of July; after a few weeks of monsoon-like rainfall, the sun has finally put in an appearance and behind me, out of the window, a bright blue sky hangs over the wader scrape. I can hear a collection of sounds coming from outside the hide, but I'm not interested in that today. If anyone wanders in through the closed door, I'm sure they will be confused to be greeted by a woman who has chosen to face away from the sights that are on offer just a few feet away.

A sound pulls me back into the room and my eyes are drawn up towards the beams that run along the length of the hide. Sitting directly above me is the now familiar figure I have spent a lot of time with this summer. The delicate frame, shrouded in shining navy feathers, clutches a white feather in its mouth, ready to line the nest that has been so carefully constructed on another beam against the outer wall of the hide.

I'll be honest, I still don't know how to tell the difference between a male and female swallow. It's something to do with the length of those iconic tail feathers. But frankly, unless I have two lined up side by side, how am I supposed to tell which tail feathers are 'short'? I'm going to guess this one is female though. Somehow, remembering this is a mother, just like me, helps me to realise that I am as much a part of the natural world as she is. After all, we aren't actually removed from nature, and despite how much we may protest, we are and always will be a part of it. We depend on it for our very survival. We aren't above nature. We aren't a distant relation of nature – we are quite literally nature. Part of the animal kingdom, mammals, members of the great ape family, with our cousins the chimpanzee, bonobo, gorilla and orangutan. We may have moved on in terms of our advanced tool use but really, at the heart of it, we are just bipedal apes. Though, sitting here in this hide with a laptop in front of me, it is difficult to believe.

It strikes me that swallows often return to the same nesting site, so could this then be the very same swallow I shared a moment with last year? My imagination wanders, thinking about the journeys we have both made in the year since we were last in this hide. Hers physical, from South Africa, risking her life to get to the breeding ground. And mine, a metaphorical journey which has taken me from some of the darkest moments of my life to the place I find myself in now, feeling brighter and somewhat happier, much like the weather.

Déjà vu strikes as I hear footsteps on the boardwalk outside, masking the chittering noise that has, until now, provided the soundtrack to this moment. The door swings open and a short woman with shoulder length, tightly curled hair, backs into the hide, hands full of camera equipment. She turns around and appears lightly startled when she spots me sitting, facing into the hide. 'Had the yellow wagtail?' she asks me briskly.

'No,' I reply, 'but there's a nesting swallow above your head,' pointing to the figure above her which somehow has not yet taken flight.

The woman ignores me and takes a seat facing out of the hide, resting her camera on the windowsill. 'Just a swallow. Seen plenty of them, don't need another one. Someone told me there was a yellow wagtail, haven't got one on my year list yet, have a look for it, will you?'

As well as her tone, her attitude immediately irritates me. It's one I have encountered countless times on nature reserves – the dismissive 'oh, it's just a ...'

It's not 'just a swallow'. It's new life forming just above our heads that we are privileged to witness.

It's not 'just a swallow'. It's a mother, gently tending to her children just as I would tend to my own and working hard for hours on end to provide them with the sustenance to allow them to grow.

It's not 'just a swallow'. It's a traveller that would shortly be embarking on a journey of life or death, across countries and continents to take tales of the Norfolk marshes to the South African landscape.

Nature is never 'just a …' Look a little bit closer and you will see even the humble woodpigeon has a story to tell if you are willing to listen. There's always more to a story, an individual, a situation, than meets the eye.

I haven't left my binoculars in the car this time, and I pull them out of my bag. Turning round, I bring them to my face and begin to scan the wader scrape. Before I could blink, a small, brightly coloured yellow ball comes into view. I watch it for a while and smile to myself: I've never seen a yellow wagtail before. This bundle of sunshine stood out amid the sea of avocets, and as I watch it hopping around, I think of how I must look on these nature reserves, usually dressed in brightly coloured floral clothing or vintage fleeces that would be at home on a 1980s ski resort. For a second, I consider telling the woman where the bird is, as I usually help anyone on a birding journey. But, just this once, the petty side of me takes control. So I stand up, pack away my things and leave the hide quietly. And yes, okay, I still feel guilty for that decision, but after all, it was *just* a yellow wagtail.

Two weeks have passed and the summer holidays have finally begun. I'm down to just one child today as the other has been deposited at his friend's house for a sleepover, cue a sleepless night as I anxiously await the 1 a.m. 'can you pick me up, please' phone call.

The local annual carnival is happening today, a huge gathering of people coming together for a chaotic day of traffic jams, crowd dodging, overpriced car parking and being conned out of an extortionate amount of money as we attempt to win poorly stitched soft toys that we could buy in Poundland.

'Do you want to go to the carnival?' I ask George, secretly praying he says no. By some miracle, he turns down the sensory overload and I (and my bank account) breathe a sigh of relief. 'What do you want to do then?' To my pleasant surprise, he replies, 'Go to the hides and see the baby swallows.'

Being the obliging parent I am, I naturally agree, and an hour later we find ourselves back at the same dimly lit wooden hide. Knowing exactly where to look, George stands up on one of the benches so he can peer into the nest that, last time he visited, was obscured by a mother who was keeping her eggs cosy underneath her warm body. To his delight, we are instead greeted by three young swallows, each one seeming bigger than the nest itself. One individual seems to have drawn the short straw, clinging on to the edge of the structure like a five-pound note glued awkwardly to the edge of a 2p slot machine, taunting the entry level gamblers as they desperately insert coin after coin in a fruitless attempt to claim victory.

The three babies sit like grumpy gremlins carved into a cathedral, wearing navy school blazers, wide mouths patiently awaiting the return of their parents. Like a preprogrammed animatronic, they turn in sync and open their mouths as the adult flies in through the window and delivers a treat into the depths of the cavernous beak of the chick at the back of the nest. As if they are part of an ornate, complex cuckoo-clock, they move in harmony back to their original places, poised to repeat the action upon their parents' next delivery.

A man walks into the hide, with various pieces of equipment slung over both shoulders, and looks at my son, who is still standing on the bench in his bright blue Crocs, excitedly peeking into the nest that he has so patiently waited to see.

'Oh hello, what have you found?' the man asks him in a friendly tone.

'Baby swallows,' George replies, gesturing towards the scene that had been playing out before us.

'Oh brilliant, this must be the second brood, wonderful! They must be nearly ready to fledge; look at that one clinging on to the edge!'

He settles himself on the bench next to us, unloading his items and immediately pointing his camera up at the nest, snapping photos and continuing to ask George questions about what else he had seen. I stand back and smile as this simple exchange takes place. An exchange that will no doubt help to shape and influence my child's experience, and encourage him on his journey as he continues to explore the natural world.

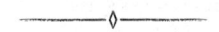

---

I find myself now sitting in a café in Holkham in June 2024. It's my favourite place on the North Norfolk coast. A lot has changed since the moment I shared with the swallow mother, but I have found myself diving deeper and deeper into the natural world and it now engulfs me and carries me through each day. Somehow, Holkham is a peaceful refuge even in the midst of the summer tourist chaos. Cars queue impatiently for the closest space to the parking ticket machine; large horses with sand coating the bottoms of their legs saunter nonchalantly, the riders unbothered by the impatient drivers. The café, a large, modern-looking wooden clad building at the end of Lady Anne's Drive car park, sticks out like a sore thumb against the backdrop of the large pines.

Behind the trees lies Holkham beach. My mind is quickly taken from peaceful images of the long, open, sandy beach when I remember a day we spent at the beach last summer, which ended with a trip to minor injuries after my son learnt the hard way why razor clam shells are called razor clam shells. I'm sitting in the undercover section of the café, making notes for this book, collecting bird stories to bring to you. My mum is sitting opposite me. She pushes her black, rectangular-framed glasses against her face as she looks down at the pages of the book she is reading. *Sex on Earth: A Celebration of Animal Reproduction* by biologist Jules Howard. She occasionally breaks away from the pages to take a sip from her boiling hot mug of English Breakfast tea or to tell me an interesting fact she's just read.

Mum is a nature lover – she's the one who encouraged my mud-centric childhood habits. We spent many days walking around the elaborate grounds of Nostell Priory, collecting daisies to make crowns and walking barefoot across the flower meadow that led back to the car park. She's a nature lover, yes, but prefers to walk and gets exasperated when I stop every thirty feet or so to whip my phone out to identify yet another leaf with Google Lens.

    A pied wagtail is staying close by, a tiny black and white clockwork toy that scuttles between the tables in the hope of a stray crumb. A familiar navy bolt makes me look up from my notebook and I follow it with my eyes up to a ledge above the café entrance. A brown basket is neatly tucked against the wall and now I know exactly what this is. I get up from my chair; Mum half glances at me but is used to me wandering off to explore, so doesn't question me. As a child, I used to escape during shopping trips and hide in rails full of clothes in Primark. Now I'm no different, only I've replaced the clothing rails with hedgerows which are packed full of treasures to behold.

    I get my phone out and use it to zoom in, getting a closer look at the nest. The adult has flown away, presumably to collect more insects for dinner, but I can see through the screen of my phone three grumpy looking faces poking out over the top. I snap a photo and laugh at the results. With their beaks closed, their scowling faces look down at me, an invader disturbing their feeding time. A couple with a freshly sheared Old English Sheepdog walk past and cast me a sideways glance, wondering what I'm doing taking photos of the doorway. They don't look up to see what I'm staring at. Curiosity doesn't get the better of them. Instead, they silently carry on into the café.

    A few more walkers pass me; not one notices the mother gliding seamlessly to and from the nest. She zooms past the eyeline of several tall men who are waiting for their partners to come out of the loos, all of them holding dogs on leads which sniff each other, tails wagging. One of them (the men, not the dogs) looks at his phone, one hand leaning on the handle of a large red pram which contains a toddler covered in mud, just how a toddler should be, I think. None of them notice. Right above their heads, there are three brand new lives developing and thriving, getting ready to face the longest journey of their lives in just a few short weeks. This astounds me for a moment, but then I remember that not even a year ago, I would have stood in this very café, too, without noticing the mother fighting to protect her family, risking her life every time she takes flight as the opportunistic buzzards circle above the open roof.

I walk back to the table and sit down, my phone open on a photo of the trio in the nest. I slide it in front of my mum. 'Baby swallows,' I say simply as she looks at the phone.

'Aw, like your grandad had,' she replies half-heartedly before continuing. Then, with a spark in her eye, she adds, 'Did you know ducks' vaginas are spiral shaped so only the male she wants can successfully mate with her?'

I may just make a birder out of her yet.

# 6
# GANNET

*'Finds tongues in trees, books in the running brooks,
Sermons in stones, and good in everything.'*
*— As You Like It*, Act 2, Scene 1

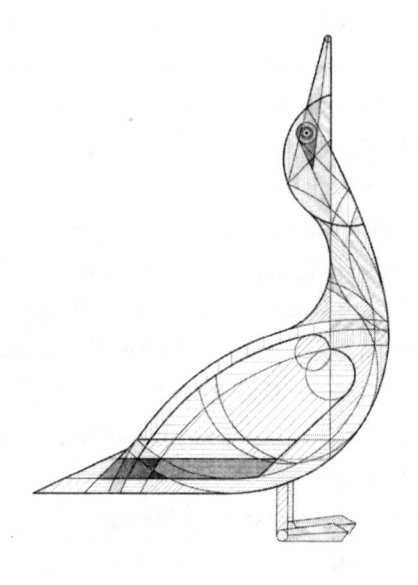

**Our fight or flight response needs a system upgrade**

If you've ever experienced that pounding heart sensation as your phone flashes up with an unknown number, or a mild inconvenience sends you into a spiral of panic, then I imagine you'll agree that our fight or flight response needs an upgrade. Designed to keep us safe from becoming someone else's prey, it now goes into overdrive if we are caught out by an unexpected knock at the door. But one bird somehow managed to teach me that there's a big world out there which will go on turning regardless of the minor hiccups that happen in our day to day lives. The gannet showed me there is so much we don't know about, so many things waiting to be discovered, and it made me realise that I am really very small in this great big world. So while I do still have a strong fight response when my pocket gets stuck on a door handle as I walk past, the gannet helped me put things into perspective and realise that I'm going to be okay, I'm not going to get eaten on the way to Asda. Honest.

———◊———

*Dolphins? What are they doing here?*

It's late afternoon in August 2023 and I've just received a text from Chris Stone to tell me that eight bottlenose dolphins have just been spotted along the coast near our house. I have to read the text several times before it sinks in, but I can't for the life of me imagine dolphins just down the road from my house.

Dolphins to me are exotic creatures of faraway waters. I've seen them on boat trips in Greece and watched my mum swim alongside them in the Canary Islands while I stayed safely aboard a boat; the depths of the ocean have never called to me. But I never, for a second, imagined they'd be near my house. But then, they live in the sea, don't they, so why not?

It's warm so it isn't hard to convince the kids to go down to the local beach to join the swarms of tourists who will be bathing in the shallows and lying uncomfortably on towels along the shingle shore, determined to enjoy the last of the evening sun, with or without sand. When we get to Cley beach, I exchange hellos with a group of birders whom I recognise from trips to local nature reserves. The kids and I walk past them and I set up my scope, pointing it in the appropriate direction where the others seem to be looking. One of the men turns around to tell me that this is a really rare occurrence, that dolphins have only ever been spotted once off this stretch of coast. So, I guess my surprise at finding out that dolphins were hanging out down the road was not unwarranted.

As I look out to the sea, one of my children lies between the legs of the tripod, wobbling it as he settles himself on the stones with his arms behind his head. The other hangs off my free arm demanding to know when it's his turn to look.

'Let me at least try and find them first, mate, give me a chance.'

'There's a dolphin. Seen it now,' he throws out casually, gesturing and then looking to where he's just pointed. And he's right. There it is, the unmistakable outline of a silvery dorsal fin and a puff of air as Flipper briefly surfaces.

Lining up the scope, I take an awkward video through the lens with my phone camera and show it to the youngest, who is still settled on the ground beneath me. It's funny weather today. Warm, yes, but looking out to sea, it's as though the elements are in a battle with themselves. The beach is framed by a pristine blue sky, the perfect picture of a summer's day with sunbathers and dog walkers relishing the moment. As though painted by a complex and conflicted artist, directly above the beginning of the water hangs a duvet of grey clouds that gradually turn darker as they head further out to sea.

The sea, to me, has always felt like a place that is not mine to explore. I attribute some of the fear I have towards it to a pretty standard human survival instinct. Some of that possibly comes from my dad chasing me round the pool singing the *Jaws* theme when I was learning to swim. That did two things: one, made me learn how to swim pretty fast and, two, ensured those two iconic notes circle around my head every time I even step a toe into the water. That said, I do fully explore the benefits of cold-water swimming and frequently find myself plunging into bodies of freezing liquid, breathing like a fish on land as I slowly acclimatise myself to the grips of the icy depths. All it takes to get me out, though, is the suggestion of a creature or some seaweed brushing against my calf. Or as happened the other day, the string off my swimming costume touching my back.

I look back at my phone screen, which I have positioned in my 'phone scope' against the lens of the scope. This allows me to turn it into a tiny TV screen and eliminates the motion sickness I feel when awkwardly squinting through the eyepiece. A large white bird glides across the phone screen, wings outstretched as it skimmed the surface of the waves. The surf reaches up as though to gently kiss the black feathers adorning the ends of the wings. I hear laughter behind me and turn to see a group of six people around the same age as me chuckling and pointing at the scope in front of me. The group is clearly departing from a day spent at the beach; one has a half-inflated rubber ring over his arm and is scrambling over the shingle, shaking pebbles out of his flip-flop every couple of steps. I remember all the times I've worn Crocs down here and spent more time emptying the stones out. They are quite obviously chuckling at the line of people here looking out to sea, no doubt perpetuating the 'birding' stereotype.

## THE LIFE-AFFIRMING MAGIC OF BIRDS

The other dolphin spectators don't seem to notice (or don't acknowledge) the group but, of course, I'm not one to miss out on an opportunity to showcase something cool, so I take a deep breath and shout towards the group, 'do you want to have a look?'

'Yeah, go on then, looking at birds?' he replies.

Without saying anything, I step back and point him towards the scope. He comes over and obligingly bends down and peers at the lens. 'Oh shit!' he exclaims. 'Is that a dolphin?!'

Immediately the rest of the group hurry forward to have a look at the spectacle unfurling before them. The dolphins continue their show, breeching and spouting water out of their blowholes in the distance as unsuspecting people paddle along the shoreline.

'Hang on,' says a woman in the group, blonde beach waves falling effortlessly over her shoulder, the kind of hair I've dreamt of having in place of the messy brunette bird's nest I've been 'blessed' with, 'we've just been swimming in the sea, so we were swimming with them!'

'Epic,' flip-flop guy returns, 'gonna tell my mates I've been swimming with dolphins.'

They thank me for showing them the incredible sight that was literally just in front of them and walk away, excitedly chattering about what they've seen. It strikes me once again that there are whole worlds out there that continue to move at the same time, whether we notice them or not. It's like that old philosophical question: if a tree falls in a wood and no one is around to hear it, does it actually make a sound? In this instance, yes, it most certainly does.

As humans, we have an obsession with ourselves and our own greatness. We are so heavily invested in our own progression and success that we ignore and forget about the millions of other species who will carry on whether or not we are around. Arguably, human success is attributed to our ability to make tools, a trait that we developed over millions of years throughout the Palaeolithic era, getting more and more complex as time went on. There's evidence, in fact, of stone tools dating back as far as 3.3 million years in Kenya and associated with our ancestors, *Australopithecus*. So, for more than three million years, we have been evolving into the dominant species, slowly (more quickly in the last couple of centuries) taking over and destroying the planet. But what would happen if you suddenly removed human tools? I don't just mean hammers and screwdrivers. I mean anything we use to 'survive' in our day to day lives. I'm talking about water filtration systems, electricity, heating, farming machinery, smartphones, books even, every tool that enables us to get 'one up' on the world around us. If we took them away, where would we be?

Perhaps we need to step back and look at the nature that flows all around us, that continues to move with little to no awareness of us humans. I often dream of becoming a swamp witch and disappearing with my family into the woods to live an off-grid lifestyle. But then I remember that without the use of my smartphone, how would I Google 'how to live off the land'? How far would I get without the tools that have made us so 'successful' as a species? Then I think, perhaps I'd better stay where I am. Yet this awareness of the world and the creatures with which we share it is what matters, to me at least. With over one million species at risk of immediate extinction because of the damage we have caused, it would serve us well to take that step back and reconnect with where we started. Perhaps then we can take a more holistic approach to wherever we are going next. The dolphins at Cley certainly don't have to Google 'how to catch a fish', so maybe they have the upper hand, or flipper. Something to ponder anyway.

So, gannets. What even is a gannet? I'll admit that I didn't know what a gannet was until relatively recently. I had my eyes opened – one of those 'what on earth is that?' moments – on a trip to Bempton Cliffs, an RSPB reserve balanced on the edge of a cliff not far from Scarborough. I'd always wanted to see a puffin and I'd read that they can often be found at Bempton Cliffs, so on a visit back to Yorkshire to see some friends, I bundled the kids into the car and started the one-hour journey from York to Bempton. And there I was introduced to a new species for me, the gannet.

———◊———

It's mid-July 2023 and I'm driving round Yorkshire. It feels comfortable; I spent most of my childhood here, growing up near Pontefract and then returning in my twenties to undertake a degree at York. If anyone ever asks me where I'm from, I suppose Yorkshire is the place that feels most familiar to me, where I spent the longest period of my life and where I have gravitated back to naturally at several points. Driving to Bempton, I'm reminded of trips I made as a child to Scarborough beach, chips by the sea with my childhood best friend, Catherine, and her wonderful family in Filey. All of the places that mean so much to me, but I am now seeing through new, fresh eyes.

# GANNET

We arrive at the gravelly car park and pull up at Bempton Cliffs to be greeted by a welcoming visitor centre. The staff on the desk try to engage the kids but after being in the car for an hour, they just want to be released into a field to run, like agility dogs in training. We hurry through a brightly lit shop and café and out on to the paths. Within a few minutes, we get a view of the perfect blue sea seemingly falling away dramatically over the steep clifftops. I can see hundreds of white shapes hovering just above the ground and assume they are gulls of some sort – my seabird knowledge isn't up to scratch just yet and, quite honestly, I have no idea what other birds could possibly be here. As we draw closer, the white shapes seem to get bigger until we are literally surrounded by them.

'What on earth are they?' I say out loud.

'Dinosaurs,' George answers simply, mimicking the way that George Pig, of Peppa Pig fame, announces his favourite animal.

I lean against the wooden barrier and look up at the birds that are encircling me. Large birds, with black tipped outstretched wings and a slight yellow tinge to their white bodies. As I watch with awe, I feel as though I have been transported inside a Christmas snow globe. The white figures are suspended on the light breeze as though held there for a moment in time. I take a snapshot with my mind and vow to remember this feeling. It's the first time I've felt properly immersed in their world. I've had my oystercatcher moment and I'm building on my knowledge of the natural world, but until now, until this moment, I've never felt part of it. This, right here, a moment shared with birds whose name I can't even tell you, is the most at peace I've felt for a very long time.

## THE LIFE-AFFIRMING MAGIC OF BIRDS

Suddenly, my eldest child shakes the proverbial snow globe by shouting across the path at me,

'GANNETS! They're gannets. Look, the baby ones are spotty like dalmatians!'

My peace, and that of everyone else in East Yorkshire no doubt, shattered, I wander over to join him at an information board which tells us everything about these birds.

'Gannet land,' Jack proclaims, giving Bempton Cliffs its unofficial nickname henceforth.

The northern gannet is an absolutely gorgeous seabird with the largest colony found here in the UK on Bass Rock in Scotland. In fact, their Latin name, *Morus bassanus*, comes from this. With their sleek plumage and slender wings, gannets are impressive figures against the backdrop of the open ocean, like pterodactyls in the opening scenes of a *Jurassic Park*. They love to snack on herring and mackerel, but to catch their prey they have a pretty impressive technique. They are the Tom Daleys of the avian world and can perform dives from heights of about thirty metres, where they soar high above the water, scanning the area for prey before folding their wings and hurtling head first into the ocean at speeds of around sixty miles per hour. To put that into perspective, an Olympic diver like Daley will reach speeds of around thirty miles per hour during a dive. Gannets obviously watched the summer Olympics diving event and thought 'double it'.

Now, imagine if you dived from thirty metres into the sea, you might be in for some nasty injuries. I don't know if you've ever jumped into a body of water but that hurts if you get it wrong. Remember playing with cornstarch as a kid, if you get the angle right, your hand slides into the liquid; get it wrong and it's hard as a brick. That's what getting a dive wrong feels like, but a bit worse. So, if you are actually an Olympic diver then you might be diving from a ten-metre diving board, but if you were an Olympian then I'd expect you would know how to employ proper techniques to minimise risk and lessen the chance of doing yourself some serious damage. Gannets saw Olympic divers with their ten-metre diving boards and thought, 'triple it'. Their streamlined bodies and specially developed air sacs beneath their skin cushion the impact of the speed, allowing them to dive to depths of over twenty metres to get their fish supper. Again, to give you some perspective, that's like travelling all the way from the top of the Leaning Tower of Pisa to the ground at sixty miles per hour.

I mentioned Bass Rock, the world's largest gannet colony and somewhere I've always wanted to visit. Imagine a big rock in the middle of the sea off the coast of Scotland. But it's so much more than a big rock. It's an entire world existing on that rock with over 150,000 gannets during the breeding season. Every inch of rock is covered in nesting birds, the air filled with the swirling confetti of white feathers as they dive in and out of the open water to take food back to their hungry babies. Oh, and those babies are worth a mention. The adult gannets are strikingly beautiful with their pristine plumage and elegant grace. Baby gannets are . . . beautiful in their own way. Imagine a gannet, but make it miniature, completely naked and a bit blue. Not sure what more I can add to that image.

Despite living the dream on the coast, gannets are listed as 'Amber' in the UK, meaning they are facing numerous threats. Pollution, overfishing and, of course, the effects of climate change are all having an impact on their food sources and, in turn, on population numbers across the colonies. The good news is there are plenty of brilliant people working to protect colonies and their habitats. Like the Scottish Seabird Centre, which continuously monitors the populations on Bass Rock. During 2023, counting the gannets was a high priority to assess the impact of the avian flu outbreak. Technological advances have introduced new tools to carry out these counts, such as drone surveys and machine learning trials.

The earliest evidence of gannets overlapping with human activity dates back thousands of years: gannet remains found in ancient coastal settlements, suggesting they may have been a food source for inhabitants. For centuries, they have been hunted for meat and eggs. Today, gannets capture the imagination of birders and are a popular subject for wildlife photographers who visit seabird colonies. With their distinctive bright blue eyes that stand out against a perfect white backdrop, it's easy to understand what has attracted people to gannets for millennia. Simon Beedie is one such photographer who's had his heart captured by the gannet. For Simon, nature is free therapy and his escape from the world. He has moderate hearing loss and tinnitus, so being able to connect visually with something offers a distraction from the bits of his brain that he describes as 'broken'.

Simon produces some of the most stunning images of gannets I've ever seen, and I ask him why he finds these birds so special. 'I mean just look at them,' he replies. 'The beautiful lines of a skypointing gannet or the crossed bills of a fencing pair of birds are so compelling to me. They've become a part of my heart and my soul.' Simon states they are the 'perfect seabird', and tells me he dreams of living near to a colony and having the time away from work to follow and capture their daily lives.

I walk with the boys along the clifftops heading further and further away from the visitor centre and into the unknown. Gannets still sprinkled in the air around us like falling confetti. Eventually, we come to a wooden viewing platform which is empty except for an RSPB volunteer who is standing with a scope and pointing something out to the colleague standing beside him. There's a gannet sitting proudly on a rocky ledge, almost within touching distance, it feels. As I watch, it looks out to sea, contemplating its next move. Then it turns towards me, and I am faced with two bright blue eyes unlike anything I've ever seen in a bird before. Not that I've spent much time staring into the eyes of birds, but these eyes are deep, replicating the ocean that gannets make an easy home from. The waves that the gannet can control as they spiral within them to catch their unwilling prey.

Another gannet lands softly next to the first and I watch as it too turns to me. This one is different. It feels different; the eyes tell a story of an experience it would rather forget. These eyes aren't blue like their companion. They're black.

While the human world was struggling with a global COVID-19 pandemic, the bird world was suffering from the effects of its own plague. High Pathogenicity Avian Influenza Virus, or bird flu, has had a negative impact for decades, but the most recent strain decimated global bird populations, and seabirds like northern gannets suffered greatly. You might remember it on the news, or signs around the local area telling people to keep chickens and ducks under cover. I spotted a sign by the lake in Bushy Park in London, advising the public to avoid feeding wild birds to help reduce the risk of spreading bird flu.

It was and still is a scary time for both the public and conservationists. A school mum and friend, Emma, has a collection of beautiful ducks that she has acquired from various places. They are very much part of her family and usually have free range of the entire large garden in the middle of the local town centre. I visited them for a coffee during the height of the bird flu outbreak, and while Emma completely understands the reason why her ducks had to be kept under cover, in line with government guidelines, it was heartbreaking for her to see her once free-running, happy ducks congregating under their new enclosure. I suppose it was not unlike our experiences of being plunged in and out of lockdown, the difference being the ducks probably have no understanding as to why they had lost access to their sprawling lawn.

During April 2022, outbreaks in Scotland, Canada, Germany and Norway saw huge numbers of dead gannets, followed by outbreaks in twelve UK and Ireland colonies. An RSPB team working on Bass Rock reported that gannet adult survival was 42 per cent lower than the previous ten-year average. A study was conducted at Bass Rock to investigate the impact of bird flu on the colony and to assess whether or not gannets were able to recover from a bird flu infection. In June 2022, black irises, instead of the usual light blue eyes, were spotted on some of the breeding gannets, and after sampling apparently healthy birds for antibodies, seven of the eight who tested positive had black irises

## GANNET

The RSPB volunteer kindly explains this to me when I ask about the bird staring at me. I'd seen the news about bird flu, I'd visited friends whose pet birds were impacted by the guidelines, but to be standing in front of this gannet who had been through the disease and come out of the other side tells a different story, a story of resilience and survival. As I stand and gaze into the black eyes of the proud looking gannet, I start to think about my own experience of the human pandemic. Of Clyde, my cousin whom we lost to Covid. It may be totally anthropomorphic of me, but I imagine the losses that this bird has suffered. A once thriving colony was almost halved by a disease that ripped through the population, but this individual has lived to tell the tale. A shared experience that brings me even closer to nature than ever before.

'—Look, Mummy, penguins!'

Brought back to earth again with a bang, I turn to George, who is standing with his head between two bars on the fence and staring down at something on the cliffs. I follow his gaze towards some birds who are resting on a ledge below us, and to the untrained eye they do indeed appear to look like miniature penguins. In fact, these birds are guillemots, seabirds and part of a family called 'auks', which, until I saw that word written down, I assumed was 'orc', and wondered why they were named after the particularly creepy characters from *Lord of the Rings*. As it turns out, a website I stumbled upon described auks as 'like penguins but can fly'. I'm certain there must be more defining features, but I quite like that one.

The guillemots we are looking at are huddled together on a protruding ledge, their white bellies perfectly outlined by a sleek black body as though it's been drawn by a stencil and a steady hand. Like gannets, they're perfectly adapted for life at sea and can propel themselves through the waves in pursuit of their prey.

As we wander back along the clifftop, hungry and in pursuit of our own prey (a cheese toastie from the café), a woman walking past with a pair of binoculars smiles and, in a Yorkshire accent that fills me with feelings of comfort, asks: 'Did you see everything you wanted?'

'No puffins today unfortunately,' I reply, disappointed but happy at the encounters I've had, nonetheless.

'Oh, you're about two weeks too late for them, most of them have left already,' she tells me.

*Brilliant*, I think to myself. It seems the iconic clown birds have eluded me for yet another summer.

———◊———

Yoav Perlman is the director of Birdlife International, Israel, an organisation dedicated to protecting the species and habitats there. I met Yoav at the Global BirdFair, which is an annual gathering of bird nerds who come together in Rutland to share their work and passions for the natural world and inspire each other. With so many people from all over the world gathering in one place for a whole weekend, it's a unique chance to meet and be inspired by people with whom our paths might never otherwise cross. It turns out that Yoav has an old friend, Mark, who lives just down the road from me in the coastal town of Sheringham, so I find myself arriving, at the end of July 2023, at a row of beautiful little cottages just a stone's throw from the smooth sea, which stretches out until it hits the perfect blue sky. I walk up to the small wooden gate that comes up to my hip height and see Yoav sitting in a white plastic garden chair on the neatly curated lawn. He smiles and says 'hello' as I spy Mark standing in his neighbour's garden, a pair of kitchen scissors in hand, trimming the straggly bits of grass around a stone bird bath. As far as first impressions go, I like Mark already.

We chat over a quick cup of very strong, fresh coffee that I already know is going to help me see through time, or at least give me jittery anxiety for the next couple of hours. It transpires that Mark has lived a fascinating life, with many years spent working and travelling all over the globe to remote corners of places I can only dream of exploring, like Papua New Guinea. His living room, a cosy space with patterned rugs, a fireplace packed with ornaments and maps around the walls, reminds me of walking into one of those heritage museums where they recreate how living rooms may have looked in the past. But this room tells a different story on every surface, each one speaking to me about a journey or an adventure, and each one building into the person Mark is today. Quite wonderful really. I know that I am in the presence of a storyteller, an unsuspecting source of information that I just want to soak up and learn from. He sends me upstairs to the landing to have a quick look at the collection of artefacts he has collected on his travels, and I am greeted by a treasure trove of stuff from intricate carvings to texts handwritten on parchment in languages I don't recognise.

It's such a beautiful day, and despite this mine of knowledge it seems a shame to spend the time together inside, so we step out into the sun and begin a steady walk along the seafront, chatting as we go about our lives. It amazes me that Mark, with all his experience and extraordinary life tales, is as interested in hearing from me about my life plans for the future. This person who could talk for weeks and probably still not have shared all of his adventures is still passionate about soaking up new information from the people around him.

I often think about this, how we as humans can be so self-centred that we think our experience is the only one that matters. We draw ourselves into arguments and debates that don't really need to be had. What if – and here is a novel idea, one which I'm not sure will catch on – instead of being sucked into arguments about which side of the fence we sit on, and I mean on every topic, whether it's conservation, politics, drama in the office, Netflix, anything. What if we actually take the time to listen to each other? I don't mean just listening and nodding along absentmindedly; I mean really *listen* and actually hear each other. So, instead of clashing heads with people who have differing views to us, we hear them and take on board what they have to say.

I only need to look on my Facebook memories that pop up daily to know how much I have changed. There's nothing more humbling than seeing angry rants that I posted twelve years ago and wondering what happened that day to trigger such one-sided and quite plainly ignorant rage. After much self-reflection, I'd like to think that I have learnt to listen to people and to learn from what they have to say. Okay, some people can't be reasoned with, but unless we start hearing each other, where are we going? We can either carry on shouting into the void of our echo chambers or we can give it a go. Can't hurt, surely?

We walk along the seafront, bypassing the high street packed full of tourists, past a freshly painted grey pub, the Two Lifeboats, that has a glass-fronted balcony. Behind the glass screen are holiday makers with half-finished pints in front of them and plates bursting with hearty meals, making me crave chips. Sunglasses on their faces, soaking up the sun. But my eyes are drawn to a line of pigeons gathered in a row above the balcony, peering over the edge to see if any crumbs have been dropped that are worth expending energy for.

'Look at those pigeons waiting for food.' I realise I've said that out loud.

Yoav smirks at me and rolls his eyes. No one seems to understand my love for the most unloved of birds. But I so love them.

One pigeon, a rainbow of purple and green shining on its back as the sun bounces off the dark feathers, makes the journey down from the rooftop on to the wall below the balcony and pecks at a piece of dried chewing gum that has been squashed into the dark bricks. It tries a couple of angles before walking along the wall and flying awkwardly into the bin in front of me. Okay, so not the kings of grace and elegance but endearing, nonetheless.

We move to the wall which sits high above the beach. Looking down at the coastal scene below, I see the tide is out and a flat, wet stretch of sand glints in the warm light of the summery day. A baby herring gull is perched, grey feathers helping it to camouflage itself among the huge rocks. It flings its head back, mouth wide, and emits a surprisingly powerful, high-pitched call. Presumably trying to summon its parents in search of its next meal. There's an adult gull over the other side of the beach which doesn't flinch at the sound, carrying on walking along the sand, spraying flecks of salt water up with each step, getting further and further away from the shouting baby bird. So, I assume that's probably one of the parents, desperately trying to grab a quick break from the persistent cry of 'I'm hungry' coming from its child.

The sea wall is adorned with colourful paintings that tell the story of the history of the area. Fishing boats and sailors' haggard faces from days spent on the choppy Norfolk seas stare back at me. A little bit further along the wall is a painting of two creatures that look very much like massive elephants on a green, grassy backdrop. It looks weird to see this painting brightening up the dull concrete wall, but there's a pretty cool story behind this image. In 1990, Margaret and Harold Hems were out for a walk on the popular tourist hot spot West Runton Beach. As they strolled along underneath the steep cliffs, they spotted a mysterious object sticking out of the cliffs. It turned out that they had accidentally stumbled upon a pelvic bone of the now extinct steppe mammoth! The following year, local fossil hunter Rob Sinclair joined the excitement when he unearthed even more mammoth bones. Naturally, an excavation ensued, led by the Norfolk Museum Service and the Norfolk Archaeological Unit and, after months of digging, they found around 85 per cent of the mammoth skeleton, making it the most complete steppe mammoth skeleton ever found in Britain.

Steppe mammoths are prehistoric titans that went extinct around 120,000 years ago. At over thirteen feet tall and weighing in at around ten tonnes, they would have towered over the more well-known woolly mammoths. They were among the largest land mammals to ever walk on the Earth, and they lived right here in Sheringham, the bustling seaside town (admittedly it would have had fewer tat shops and cafés back then). Can you imagine, a casual walk on the beach leading to such an amazing find? This only further validates the thing I keep going on about: if you open your eyes and start paying attention to your surroundings, you may just spot something incredible. Okay, it might not be a mammoth skeleton, but other cool discoveries are available and waiting for you.

Leaning against the wall, Yoav lifts his binoculars up to his eyes and watches the sea for a moment. Mark pulls a pair of vintage binoculars seemingly out from nowhere and copies his action, and I look out across the waves in the general direction they are pointing (my bins are in the car, obviously).

Some clouds have rolled in over the sea and there is rain in the distance. Grey clouds falling in wisps like the dementors closing in on Harry Potter, their cloaks trailing and vanishing into nothing. The sea has changed too, reflecting the mood of the sky, and matches the colour of a dark pair of jeans worn by a passer-by. Looking out across the water, I watch gulls glide past and remember what Yoav had said to me about his connection with nature. He told me that nature is his safe place, where he feels most at peace with himself. Right now, I know exactly what he means. Have you ever just stood and looked out across a body of endless water? No phones, no noise, just you and the vast expanse.

Yoav pokes me on the arm with the end of his binoculars and then points with them, 'Look at the bottom of that wind turbine, there's a gannet passing through.'

## THE LIFE-AFFIRMING MAGIC OF BIRDS

Taking the binoculars and zooming myself into where he was gesturing, I see the ghostly white figure sail through the lens of the binoculars and disappear, blending into the haze of the ocean. The bird I had only discovered earlier this month was now here in my local town. Once again, I find myself having one of those moments, surprised to have had a particular nature encounter. Perhaps I don't spend enough time staring at the sea. Perhaps I don't know enough about the wildlife in this area. Yet seeing a gannet pass by so effortlessly has filled me with that peace Yoav talked about so fondly.

Until relatively recently, I'd never heard of a gannet. So that means for about twenty-eight years of my life, these birds were going about their business, being so beautiful on the clifftops, just an hour from where I'd spent a large portion of my childhood, and I didn't even know it. If there are birds so close to home that I've never heard of, then what else is out there waiting for me to discover? It makes me realise how tiny we humans actually are in this world. While the impact we manage to have collectively on this planet is massive, in the grand scheme of things, from where I am sitting right now, you and me are pretty small.

Sometimes, if I'm having what feels like the worst day imaginable, I take myself to the sea and look out at the vast expanse and imagine the worlds that exist beneath the waves, some of them not even known to science. After all, we know more about space than we do about what's down there. Some days, when sitting behind the laptop gets a bit much, I look out of the window at the busy sparrows in the hedge which keep working to build their nests, collect food and raise their own broods. They don't care that my Microsoft Teams isn't working once again or that I've got heightened anxiety over a looming deadline. Our quest for survival is just as real as our ancestors who lived alongside the steppe mammoth, who hunted for food and crafted tools to use. Our desire to do well is no different to that of the sparrows raising their chicks. Our journey through this modern world just looks a bit different now. Our fight or flight response which was designed to help us evade becoming prey, or fight to live in a world without advanced technology, is still there. It seems we didn't get the memo that we aren't likely to be eaten by a now extinct predator or trodden on by a mammoth on the way to Asda (other supermarkets are available). The fear that hits us when an unknown number flashes up on the screen needn't cause such heightened emotions, and yet it does. An unexpected knock at the door should not fill us with absolute dread, but for some reason it often does. Fight or flight is supposed to save us from immediate danger, not from an unsolicited call from our colleagues.

I want to highlight that this time I'm not talking about major life traumas or huge life-altering events; I'm just talking about those minor inconveniences that occur for every one of us daily. Our kids forgetting their coats at school, a misunderstanding between us and our partners, an extra task being added to our daily work pile. So, I suppose the point I keep coming back to is that those gannets taught me the world will always go on turning, and all of the people, animals, plants in it will go on surviving. So, I guess I need to find a way to do that, too. Is nature the answer?

# 7
# HERRING GULL

*'But I am now about no waste; I am about thrift.'*
– The Merry Wives of Windsor,
Act 1, Scene 3

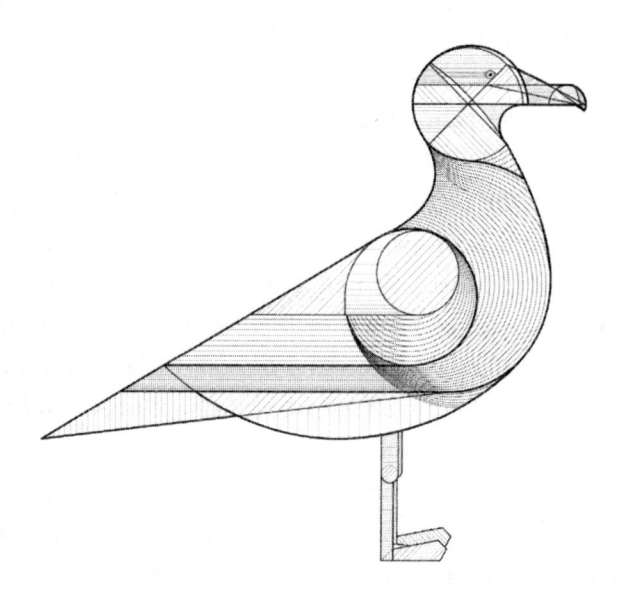

**Nature teaches us the power of resilience**

It's almost midway through 2021, the world is just emerging from the life-changing events of the previous year, and I know that I need to make a change.

After completing a degree at the University of York, largely from the kitchen table as we were thrown in and out of different levels of lockdown, I'd been about ready to break. Navigating a world where it was considered normal to

# HERRING GULL

stockpile loo roll, bake banana bread until we never wanted to look at another banana again, stand on the doorstep clapping for key workers while the government played by their own rules, I've decided it's time to take action in my own life for the sake of my mental health and my children. I was in a financial pit, barely scraping through, resorting to food banks, but I was determined to graduate and set my life on a new course, and I did. At this time, I hadn't met my oystercatcher yet; I hadn't had that single moment that set me on a different path, but I am about to have an experience that will contribute to that change. I just can't see it at this time.

I've always been drawn to mountains, particularly the mountains of North Wales. I have an entire childhood full of memories of hiking up Snowdon with my parents, swimming in Llyn Padarn or exploring the slate quarries which stand high above the towns. So, one day, I made the very spontaneous decision to move there. As you do. It felt at the time the right choice to continue my education and pursue a masters degree. I've moved around a lot all of my life so moving again didn't faze me. My children were young enough to move without affecting their schooling, and though I had barely scraped through my degree financially, I really needed to make a change to our lives. I found a private landlord who rented to students and was fortunate enough to find a rental property that was cheaper than the York equivalents. So, feeling very much like a Georgian woman being sent to the seaside to cure her hysteria, I've relocated myself and my two very young children to the coastal town of Bangor. Now, I'm not known for thinking about my plans. I've always been very much an 'act now work it out later' kind of person, but I think this was probably the most extreme I've ever pushed this personality trait. Luckily, this chaotic decision paid off and despite some hiccups, it ended up being one of the best things to ever happen to me. In this chapter, we're going to find how much nature teaches us about resilience, human and otherwise.

---◊---

It's May and I've lived in Wales for a week now. It's been a whirlwind of unpacking boxes and trying to get to grips with the layout of our new town. I've spent a day screwing together IKEA units and trying to find a place for all of the tat I seem to have accumulated during my many house moves over the last few years. There's a cupboard under the stairs where most of the boxes are being stored and, I predict, will remain there until we move again. I sit down at the kitchen table and watch a white bubble on top of my coffee cup twirl around the liquid as I remove the spoon. A movement out of the window grabs my attention, and I look up to see a very large white bird sitting on the green wheelie bin, staring menacingly through the window directly at me. Amused, I call my mum in to look, and as she runs in, I expect the gull's wings to flap and take off at the disturbance; instead, it stares at me for a long second before hopping on to the top of the black bin. Using it as a platform, it tears open a bin bag which is sticking out of the green bin. I glance up at the industrial grey fence and see another gull peering down, waiting to see if its friend comes up with the goods.

I'm leaving the kids with my mum this morning as I'm going to meet with my new supervisor. I'm giving postgraduate study a go at the University of Bangor this

September. It will later transpire that doing a masters by research straight after coming out of a pandemic probably wasn't the right decision at the time, especially as a masters loan only covered the fees and, with two children and rising childcare costs, I was unable to work enough to make ends meet. Financial accessibility to academia is a topic for another day, but it was painful to admit that I wasn't able to continue with this dream, and yet it brought us to Wales and that turned out to be great for all of us for other reasons.

Dr Alex Georgiev is a great character. He is a primatologist who directs the Zanzibar Red Colobus Project, which researches the effect of human-induced change in red colobus monkeys. I'm often greeted on Instagram by his images of the paradise-like locations he travels to, white sand beaches and turquoise seas, on his research trips. We meet at the front of the university and begin the climb upwards through the grounds. I soon realise how unfit I have become when I find myself breathing heavily as Alex, with his long stride, pulls himself effortlessly up the hill. It's hard to have a conversation when you're trying to gasp for air and also conceal the fact that you're desperately out of shape. I think the pink cheeks probably give it away.

We arrive at a footpath which runs along the top of the city. It's peaceful up here, a tarmac path that's lined with trees that create a shelter from the sun and give me a chance to cool down from the exertion. Alex gestures across the Menai Strait, a stretch of water separating mainland Wales from Anglesey, and begins pointing out landmarks.

'That's a peaceful sound,' I say, listening to a bird in one of the trees as we walk.

## THE LIFE-AFFIRMING MAGIC OF BIRDS

'Blue tit,' Alex says in his trademark direct manner. It turns out Alex is a keen birder, one of those people who can recognise birdsong from a single note, or so it seems.

I've never really thought about birdsong before. I've never considered that individual birds perform to create the cacophony of music that greets me every time I'm outside. I've never really noticed it at all. Alex tells me that he's been learning birdsong for years, and after I express a wish to be able to recognise individual bird calls, he assures me that anyone can do it, that it just takes practice.

I remember feeling in awe of his ability as he talked to me about birds and their song, hearing his passion, and realising again how much was out there that I'd never noticed before. I recall wondering how I'd never considered what might be making the beautiful calls I came to hear every morning, or what was shouting from the treetops as I went for daily walks during lockdown. When I think about that, it's Alex who began to open my eyes up to the birds around me. He gave me the key to open the door myself. All it took was someone to stand with me and unveil a world that had always been right in front of me, but which I was too blinkered to see. And that is what I hope to share with you now in this book. For me, Alex stands out as one of the pinnacle moments in my journey to reconnecting with nature. It wasn't long after our walk that I met my oystercatcher, propelling me and my children down the rabbit hole of the natural world, and discovering endless possibilities along the way.

―――◊―――

## HERRING GULL

The Llanberis Path is one of six main routes up Snowdon, the highest mountain in Wales or, as it's officially known, Yr Wyddfa. It's often cited as the most boring of the routes but I disagree. The main thing to know about the Llanberis Path is, in my opinion, it's bloody steep. And so, for the first time in my life, I am standing at the beginning of the path, a large backpack stuffed with supplies that I most likely won't need, ready to climb a mountain by myself.

This is what I moved to Wales for. I knew somehow that having the opportunity to spend my time in the great outdoors surrounded by vast mountains would be the therapy I needed to pull me out of the hole I found myself in post degree and post pandemic. I've got a very busy mind; there's always noise happening up there. It baffled me to find out that not everyone has an internal monologue. I struggle to understand how there are people out there who don't have verbal thoughts running through their heads. Inside my mind is like a tube station at rush hour, with a marching band thrown in for good measure. I can have full conversations with myself in the voices of people I'm having imaginary conversations with; I can play the entire theme to *Jurassic Park* with all the individual instruments. Negative thoughts are allowed to swirl around in there, uncontrolled and unstoppable.

I drag myself up the very steep beginning of the path, pulling myself up the slope and away from the town, getting higher and higher as my breathing becomes more and more laboured. Stepping through an iron gate that squeaks as I heave it towards me, I turn around and realise there is not a soul in sight. I stare back at the town below and realise I am truly alone. Climbing for around an hour, my thighs beginning to ache more with every step. Why on earth am I putting myself through this?

The path levels out as I reach what is, according to the instructions on my phone, the halfway point, my destination. There are some dark clouds rolling in in the distance; it seems as though the mountain is warning me not to carry on any further. I stop and sit on a large rock which is set to the side of the path. A runner appears from nowhere wearing only a light yellow T-shirt, bright red shorts and trainers. He effortlessly leaps from stone to stone along the path, like a sugar plum fairy as he bounds down the mountain.

I open my bag and pull out a sandwich that I stuffed in there this morning. The cheese is sticking out awkwardly and there's a water bottle-shaped dent in the middle of the stodgy white bread. Not my finest culinary endeavour, admittedly, but it's not a bad view to dine in. From here, I can see what feels like an endless scene of slate-covered mountains; grassy fields grazed by sheep interject at sporadic points along the way. A light drizzle taps at my face, and I pull the hood of my waterproof coat over my head. I'm standing up now, taking in the view from an elevated position before realising something: my mind is silent. The raucous noise that usually fills the gap between my ears is empty. My only thoughts are of the moment, the stillness and the clarity I'm experiencing from up here. I know at that moment that this was the right decision, moving here; removing myself from the stresses of my former life was potentially life-saving. I realise how well I feel, how much lighter, as though a weight has been lifted from me. I'm healing and this is just the start of the journey

## HERRING GULL

and I know that I've found my therapy. In nature, I've found my peace.

A black-headed gull lands on a rock next to me, looking out over the view. I throw the remains of my squashed sandwich towards the bird and it swoops to get it gratefully, swallowing up the crust before landing back on the rock, watching me, beckoning me to step into its world.

And stepping into its world is exactly what I have done.

So, let's talk about gulls. Seagulls, bin chickens, rats with wings, whatever you know them as, I'm sure you'll agree these birds have a bit of a bad rep. Imagine a seagull and I can almost guarantee that the bird you're thinking of is actually a herring gull. This large, white-headed bird with grey wings and a yellow beak with a trademark red spot at the end is a popular seaside image. Herring gulls are one of the most widespread and recognisable seabirds and can be found in around seventy countries in the northern hemisphere. They've managed to cement themselves into our towns and cities, and have become an integral part of coastal ecosystems and of our beloved seasides.

In properly wild settings, they can be found in a range of habitats including beaches and cliffs, and their breeding colonies are often found on offshore islands, living alongside other species like the well-loved puffin or aforementioned gannet. Despite their widespread distribution, herring gulls face a number of challenges that have led to them being placed on the UK Red List for species of serious conservation concern. One of the main reasons for their dramatic population drop is, once again, the human impact on their landscape. Habitats have been lost as we encroach on their territory, replacing their nesting sites with buildings, their feeding grounds with fish and chip shops. Human aversion to these gulls is mainly down to their seemingly often aggressive scavenging behaviour. How many times have you been on the beach and had a swarm of gulls after you for one thing and one thing only: your chips? But think about it: imagine someone moved into your house, built a new one on top of it and took away your favourite restaurant. You'd have to look for an alternative solution and this is exactly what gulls have done.

They've shown incredible adaptability and resilience, with some populations turning from clifftop nesters to city centre aficionados, honing in on areas where human food waste is in abundance. It might be a big ask, but I'm here to ask you to give gulls a chance. It's not their fault and, if anything, we should be impressed at their tenacity and desire to survive. Yes, okay, it's not ideal when you get a fearless and quite large dinosaur landing on the pub table and nicking your food, but can you imagine a seaside scene without herring gulls? I certainly can't.

I'm ashamed to admit but once, not so long ago, I was firmly entrenched in the 'hating seagulls' camp. After being pooed on and terrorised on the beach in Scarborough as I tried to eat my lunch, I would definitely not have called myself a gull lover. Then I moved to Wales. I saw the same two gulls (I'm convinced they were the same ones, anyway) landing on my bins every morning in search of supplies. I watched as they would throw back their heads, bills wide open as they called that iconic call across the street. I wondered how they managed to look so menacing and full of expression without eyebrows. I developed a rapport with those birds and looked forward to opening the blinds and seeing them every morning. I'm not ignoring the mess they make in towns and cities. Some mornings, the walk to school would involve dodging around the contents of bin bags that had been ripped open, sprawled across the pavements. One morning, a text from the school came through asking parents to bring the children through the back door instead of across the main playground, as a pair of gulls were dive bombing passers-by and they didn't want any children to be injured by the birds. But in reality, all those gulls were doing is what I do every day, protecting their children. Ripping open bin bags wasn't a way of inconveniencing disgruntled locals; it was their way of simply trying to survive. And isn't that what we are all trying to do? It's never too late to learn about something you misunderstand. Who knows, you may just discover something that changes the way you see the world around you.

———◊———

Sefton Park is a 200-acre green space in the heart of Liverpool. It's a busy area with people using it as a cut through on their commute and with families enjoying the opportunity to be away from urban life for a while. It's June 2023 and the park really is a brilliant green space. Wildflower verges have been left to grow along paths that run alongside tower blocks of flats, and the large lake which acts as the centrepiece is filled with wildlife living harmoniously alongside the locals. Designed by Édouard André, it opened in 1872, and around every corner you can see evidence of its Victorian roots, from the sweeping lawns to the tree-lined avenues. At the heart of the park is the Palm House, a large glass conservatory which contains a collection of exotic plants from all over the world, a botanist's heaven, and there's also a café that does really good cake. I'm here with my mum, who, having grown up in Liverpool, recounts her memories of Sefton Park from childhood. She tells me about all the times she would walk with her cousins, Joe and Dave, and their dog, Lassie (classic dog name), through the park. I remember Joe speaking with humour about the time my mum rescued him and Dave from a group of skinheads. She is tiny but you wouldn't mess with her so I can believe this story, although the image makes me laugh.

We are standing looking at a small body of water which feeds back into the main lake. There's a coot that is busy collecting nesting materials, carrying them back and forth to its partner sitting on top of a nest, presumably guarding some eggs.

'Here y'are. Look,' an unfamiliar voice with a strong Scouse accent comes from behind and I turn round to see a man of about seventy, wearing grey trackie bottoms and a black bomber jacket, beckoning me towards the other end of the water we are looking at. He leans his rickety bike against a tree and walks to where he wants me to look.

Obligingly, I follow him and he squats down, pulling out a small bag of duck food from his jacket pocket. A high-pitched clucking sound comes from the reeds and a moorhen paddles its way eagerly towards him. They are like two old friends greeting each other. The bird seems to have been waiting for him.

'She's got a nest there, not long, and the babies will be popping out to get some of this.' He gestures to the duck food he is now sprinkling in front of the moorhen, which gobbles it up quickly before disappearing back towards the nest (now obvious since he's pointed it out).

When will I develop my observational skills?

Moorhens are actually really cool water birds that you will know, most probably, from your local park. They have mainly black bodies, like coots, but where coots have a white patch on the top of their heads, moorhens instead have a red bill, the colour blending into their plumage. They have the weirdest feet. Perfectly adapted to their watery habitat, they have three 'toes' which point forward, but each one has what can only be described as lobes that join together to form propellers helping them to navigate the water. Oh, yeah, and their legs are yellowy green, standing out against the black bodies as though someone has picked up the parts of several different birds, stuck them together and thought, 'that'll do'. They are master builders and construct floating nests made out of reeds and grasses before sharing egg incubation and parenting duties. The best bit about moorhens is the fact that whether you're by a pond in rural Norfolk or a lake in the middle of Liverpool, you can spend time with these birds. You, too, can marvel at their freaky feet.

The man continues to sprinkle the food into the water and two mallards hurry towards him so as not to miss out on the prize. It really does feel as though all the birds here know him personally and feel comfortable in his presence.

'Do you spend a lot of time here?'

'Only every day for the last sixty years,' he replies. 'Used to walk along this path to me school, then to work every morning; now I come here every day to feed the ducks. I'm on my own so it gets me out and it's nice to have a chat if someone will listen. People don't seem to stop as much now though.' This is said light-heartedly, but I can sense the loneliness in him.

We keep chatting and he tells me about the moorhens, how he has watched moorhens nesting here for years. He points out a bird to me I've never seen before, diving in and out of the water effortlessly, a little grebe that looks like a small current bun.

'There was a heron last year that landed there and ate one of the babies.' He's pointing at the little grebe which has just disappeared beneath the surface again. 'There's a fish in there that was released years ago. Goldfish, big orange thing. It's still alive and it's about that big now,' he gestures the size of the fish with his hands, and though unconvinced, I encourage him.

'You seem to know all of the wildlife in the park!' I say, genuinely thrilled with this interaction and the insight into the local nature goings on of this city centre oasis.

'No, I don't know much at all. Couldn't tell you anything useful about any of the birds. I just come here every day and love watching them. This swan's my mate,' he says as a large male swan wanders over to him like a child running excitedly to an ice cream van they know is fully stocked. 'He always comes to say "hello", don't you.' The swan looks like it might actually be listening to him.

It's wonderful to be in the company of this man, who spends every day with these birds and can tell me anecdotally about each one of them. A living embodiment of the fact that you don't need to be an expert to be passionate about and interested in what's on your doorstep. He has spent sixty years walking through the park every day on his way to school, then work, then with his family and now, in the late autumn of his life, alone. He could have walked through every day, blinkers on, paying no attention to the species that he passed by each time, but instead, he chose to open his eyes and connect with the nature around him. This connection has provided him with something special, a little escape every day. He tells me that coming to the park and sitting with the birds is like spending time with friends and I think that is beautiful. Wouldn't it be wonderful if we all saw our surroundings like that and considered the species we share our spaces with as friends? Would the world look different if, instead of treating wildlife with indifference, we embraced them and welcomed them into our lives?

Well, it's never too late.

———◊———

August 2023, and it's hot today, probably a bit too hot for my liking to be outside, walking up a gentle slope that feels like a mountain as the sun beams down on my bare arms. I'm in Wiltshire visiting my dad, and a visit to Dad is never complete without a stop off at a location with some kind of historical significance. Wiltshire, a county in the west of England, definitely isn't short of historical locations.

The path leading up to West Kennet Long Barrow is wide and covered in a carpet of lush, springy, green grass. With five-foot tall rapeseed plants filling the fields on either side, it's as though someone has parted the field in the middle to provide access up to the Neolithic burial chamber. Dating back around five thousand years, and tucked into the rolling Wiltshire hills, West Kennet Long Barrow stands as a reminder of the deep, ancient spirituality that can be felt all over this area. It's one of the most impressive and well-preserved burial chambers in Britain, holding fifty individuals, buried or cremated, before the chambers were blocked up.

Archaeologists, first in 1859 and again in 1955, have uncovered the remains of males, females, adults and children as well as artefacts associated with burials from the Neolithic period such as pottery, beads and stone tools. The site's location links up with other significant sites from similar time periods such as Avebury and Silbury Hill. It speaks of the ceremony and spiritual significance our ancestors placed on life and death and makes my mind whirl, wondering who these people were, and why they decided to build such a carefully constructed set of chambers here. Did they feel the same as we do when we attend a funeral today?

I remember learning about a 50,000-year-old Neanderthal excavation in Shanidar Cave in Iraq, where archaeologists found what looked like a deliberate burial site, with evidence of flowers. Imagine that. A now extinct species of human, whose DNA we still carry with us, exhibiting the same funeral behaviours we see today across cultures. We may have moved on technologically, but underneath all of that, humans are still the same vulnerable, sensitive animals which we have been since our evolutionary journey began. West Kennet Long Barrow seems to me a reminder of the human quest for meaning and a connection with something bigger than ourselves.

Walking up the wide grassy path, the smell of the rapeseed flowers hit my nose, the scent filling me with summer vibes. My dad, who in his usual fashion is powering off ahead of the group, sneezes loudly and I assume he doesn't have the same feeling towards the bright blooming flowers as I do.

## HERRING GULL

The kids run off ahead to catch Grandad as I linger behind, stopping to take a photo of a bee resting on a large leaf, and then squeal as the bee takes flight in my direction. A couple in matching raincoats give me a sideways glance as they walk past, curious to know what caused that horrid noise to escape my lips. A swallow swoops over the path, directly in my eyeline, and I call to the kids: 'A swallow nearly hit me in the face.' They turn to see as another dives across the path.

This sea of flowers seems to be the perfect meeting point for insects, unwittingly creating the ultimate buffet for the swallows which soar with little effort across the fields on either side of the path, skimming the tops of the flowers and scooping up the unsuspecting insects. I hear a noise that grabs my attention and seems to get louder and louder. Do you remember back in the day (showing my age) when you'd sit at the computer and attempt to connect to the internet? A box would appear on the screen showing the various stages of connection and the 'dial-up tone' would ring out for the computer's tinny speakers. The AOL dial-up tone, if you can't recall, was a distinctive sound that began with a series of quick, high-pitched electronic chirps and beeps, overlapped by a collection of whirring sounds as the modem connected to the service provider. You'd also hear that sound if you picked up the landline when someone was connected to the internet. Your mum picking up the phone to ring your grandma could ruin an internet browsing session, cutting it off unexpectedly as the connection could only handle one thing at a time. The internet dial-up sound coming from the field takes me back to sitting in the family office room, surrounded by hairy dogs and piles of paperwork, as I played on Neopets, downloaded dodgy files from Limewire, filled the computer with viruses we didn't really understand and conducted homework research on Encarta. This sound, though, is made by a skylark.

Skylarks, with their modem melodies, embody, for me at least, the beauty and wonder of the natural world. These enchanting birds have inspired poets, musicians and nature lovers for centuries. Skylarks are also known for their aerial acrobatics display, and during the breeding season male skylarks ascend into the sky in a series of daring displays, soaring to great heights before descending in a fluttering cascade. I encountered my first skylarks while sitting on a North Norfolk beach. The dial-up tone rang out from the cliffs above me and I looked up to see a tiny dot spiralling upwards into the sky. Lottie Glover, bird lover and conservationist, whom I was spending the day with, seeing my curiosity peaking, pointed upwards and cried, 'Oh, skylarks!'

From that moment on, I have revelled in the sound every time I hear it. It's another one of those noises that I can't believe I went without noticing for so many years of my life. And now it's so known to me, I can't miss it.

Finally joining my family at the top of the hill, I'm slightly overheated but smiling at the beautiful encounters I have had on the way up. A quintessential English scene greets me as I look out over fields, bright sunshine yellows and fifty shades of green wave back at me as the undulating landscape unfolds. The kids run off to explore the burial chamber, the little one stopping to call for me before he walks into the dark tunnels. Looking for reassurance.

'Did you hear those skylarks?' I ask my dad as we follow the children in the footsteps of our ancestors.

## HERRING GULL

'Yeah, sounded like the internet connecting,' he replies, and I laugh at the fact that we are on the same wavelength.

A herring gull lands on top of the entrance to the chamber. I picture a map of the UK and imagine where Wiltshire sits. West Kennet Long Barrow must be at least fifty miles from the sea. These naturally coastal birds are swooping in on inland urban areas and laying claim to them. I probably wouldn't think twice if I saw a gull in the middle of Birmingham, but now that I think about it, Birmingham is 120 miles from the nearest coastline so that's even more bizarre than seeing a gull in Wiltshire. Distribution of gull species, often herring gulls and black-headed gulls (the ones you're most likely to see as you do your high street shopping), has changed a lot over the last half a century. Birds are moving inland to breed; some are feeding exclusively in these new terrestrial environments. These species, along with many others who have displayed stark changes in habitat and behaviour, could have collapsed. But they haven't. They have demonstrated a kind of real time evolution. Usually, it takes millennia to occur, but many species have shown us dramatic alterations in just a few generations. They have illustrated that, despite the pressure we have put on them, destroying their habitats, removing their nesting sites and reducing their opportunities to feed in their natural habitats, they have adapted. Their resilience in the face of adversity is something that, in my view at least, should be admired. Perhaps we should take a leaf out of their book. It seems funny to see seabirds this far inland, but I guess it shows their adaptability once again.

The gull throws back its head and sings its song, calling loudly into the wind.

# THE LIFE-AFFIRMING MAGIC OF BIRDS

———◊———

Sitting on the windswept shores of West Runton Beach, it's September 2023, and I've got an annual parking pass and I'm trying to make the most of it. The breeze tousles my already knotty hair and I savour the serenity of the shore. I've just dropped the kids at school and the only person I've seen this morning here is a man walking his excitable Cockapoo, which ran over to greet me with a kiss. I feel a sense of contentment wash over me, relishing the simple pleasure of sitting by the sea. When we left Wales, I was heartbroken. But we made up for it by ensuring we relocated to another coastal location so I could still enjoy the peace that I had found by living in such close proximity to the open waves.

I don't normally eat bananas, the texture makes me want to gag, but I haven't been shopping for a week and this was the only thing I could find in the house to grab as a breakfast to go. As I peel back the slightly brown skin of the banana, not particularly eager to tuck in, I notice a lone herring gull wandering along the sand nearby, its keen side eye fixed on my food.

Jokingly (at this point I feel I may finally have gone mad), I hold the banana out to the gull and ask, 'Would you like some, it's minging so you're welcome to it?' I laugh, amused by the idea of sharing my breakfast with a feathered friend. The gull looks at it but keeps walking along until it's out of sight. I'm not surprised that it didn't take me up on such a prize.

I keep watching the waves, thinking about the tasks that are on my 'to do' list today. The banana, the texture of which really isn't inviting, hangs limply as my hand rests on my

## HERRING GULL

knee. Then out of nowhere, in one seamless motion, a flap of wings forces a cold draught on my skin and a chunk of the banana is snaffled. The thief lands a few feet away from me and I watch on as it tries to get the now mushed banana to slide down its throat. A few failed attempts and the banana chunk is spat out on the sand where it lays discarded and unwanted. The gull looks triumphant regardless and gives me its trademark menacing glare. I can't suppress a quiet laugh at the audacity of the bird; its gumption is impressive. Once upon a time, a gull on a beach nicking my food would have sent me into a flap, squealing as the dragon attacked, or so it would seem. Now, I can't help but admire them. They are masters of adaptability, and all they are trying to do is survive.

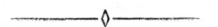

———◊———

There are seven different species of gull that regularly breed here in the UK. The herring gull of seaside fame, the chip-eating black-headed gull, the lesser black-backed gull of supermarket rooftops, the greater black-backed gull that I've spotted along the beach in Great Yarmouth, common gulls, which I'm not convinced I've ever actually seen, the mediterranean gull which, to me, looks the same as a black headed gull (sorry bird nerds) and the kittiwake, so-named because of the call they make from their clifftop nests but who are also seen in abundance nesting in various parts of Scarborough town centre. All of them are wonderful in their own unique way, and each brings with them evidence of resilience and adaptability in the face of human interference.

High above the busy car park of Kings Lynn Tesco sit a group of lesser black-backed gulls. With dark grey wings and piercing stare, these gulls are a familiar sight to the shoppers below, perched atop the supermarket's sign, surveying their domain with a watchful gaze. For these gulls, the rooftop of Tesco is much more than just a vantage point or a place to rest. It is a sanctuary amid the chaos of the town below. From their safe perch, they can observe the comings and goings of the world below, the endless stream of cars, the flow of rush hour traffic, the swarms of caravans passing through on their way to their coastal holiday destinations, pedestrians wheeling their trolleys stacked full of food for their weekend barbecues. The lesser black-backed gulls aren't just passive observers here. They have made the rooftop their own personal hunting ground, scouring the surrounding area for scraps of food and discarded treats. Waiting like vultures for a meal deal to be tossed aside or a child to drop a crisp. With their keen eyesight and sharp beaks, they are adept at spotting opportunities in among the chaos of the urban landscape, whether it be a half-eaten slice of cake left on a bench or a forgotten pack of chips from the nearby McDonalds tossed out of the car by a careless passer-by. The supermarket gulls have carved out a comfortable niche for themselves here on the roof, finding solace in the simple pleasures of food and freedom.

So, next time you're on the beach or in a busy town centre and you spot a gull, take the time to look at it and get to know it. Look into their expressive faces and find out about their individual characters. Whether they are a kittiwake nesting on a remote clifftop alongside the elegant gannets, or a lesser black-backed gull sitting on the roof of your local Tesco, cut them a bit of slack. It's not their fault; they're just doing what they need to do to get through the day.

Instead of resenting their presence, think about the real time evolution that's happening as we continue to destroy their natural habitats. They are constantly displaying inspiring levels of resilience, adapting to situations that we have forced them into.

Get to know them. And remember, it's never too late to have your mind changed. It's never too late to learn.

# 8
# CURLEW

*'And now let's go hand in hand, not one before another.'*
— Comedy of Errors, Act 5, Scene 1

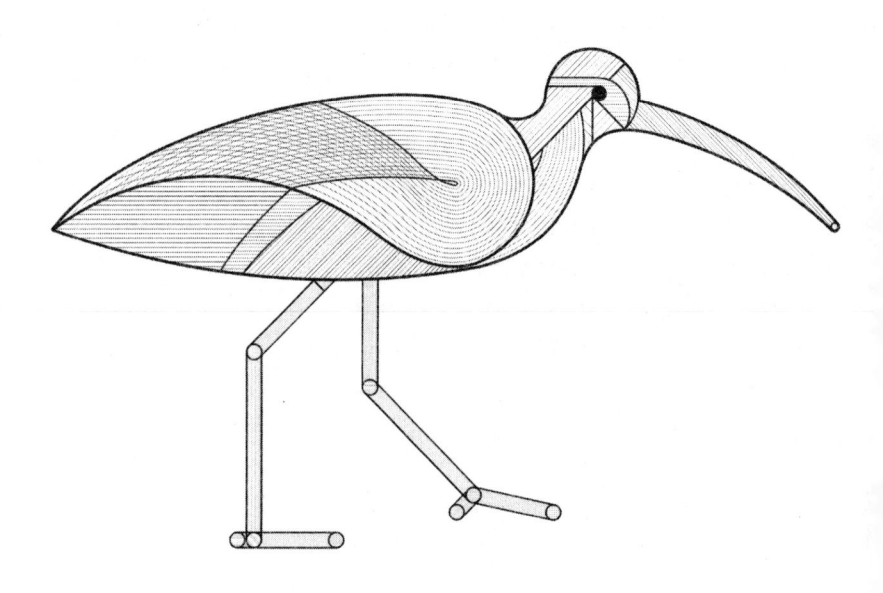

**Never lose that sense of wonder**

I realise, as I try to persuade you that nature is actually really cool and encourage you to discover your own bird story, most of this book is my journey. My stories. My life and my experience. But what about the stories of other people who have connected with nature in their own ways and, in some cases, made their own bird story the centre to their whole existence?

## CURLEW

So, this chapter is dedicated to other people and the positive effects that birds have had on them, starting with Mary.

Every person on this Earth has their own story, but Mary Colwell is particularly remarkable. Upon meeting Mary, you're greeted with warmth and genuine interest, but you soon realise that under the surface is a strong force, a storm that is churning up change for one particular bird. The curlew. Mary is the director of Curlew Action, a charity dedicated to one of nature's most pressing conservation concerns: the plight of the curlew.

The curlew isn't a bird that you will generally be able to see from your doorstep. They are large wading birds which blend into their surroundings. In summer, they can be found nesting inland, usually in farmland and uplands where they breed, and, in winter, you can spot them on coastal mudflats and estuaries. Their scientific name, *Numenius arquata*, means, respectively, 'new moon' and 'bow shaped'. The latter refers to the shape of their large bill, which curves out and down and makes them recognisable and iconic in a landscape. While you may not be able to see them from your own back garden or city centre location, they're a bird that seems to transcend the boundaries of what we expect from nature, bringing something magical and mystical with them, and an encounter with them is like meeting a mysterious old friend from a forgotten time.

Like many people I've had the pleasure of meeting during research for this book and beyond, Mary wasn't always 'into nature'. She grew up on the outskirts of Stoke-on-Trent, near the Peak District. This makes me think of Chet, our swift rehabilitator who also spent a lot of years in the Peaks. Maybe there's something about the place that subliminally shows people the wonder of the natural world without them even realising.

Nature was always present in Mary's life. She remembers walks with her dad, who wasn't particularly good at ID'ing things but noticed nature and appreciated the magic. He would comment on natural occurrences in the garden: the badger who dug up the grass, the melanistic grass snake in the compost heap, the disappearance of cuckoos and lapwings that used to be so common. Nature wasn't a major part of Mary's youth; it was always there but it wasn't a focus. It wasn't until she worked with the BBC's Natural History Unit that her eyes were opened to the vastness of the wild world, and she decided she wanted to do something to have a positive impact on its future. Mary found herself enchanted by curlews, the way they moved, their behaviour, their sound, and this pressed her to want to do something to protect them. I suppose it's fair to say that curlews are to Mary what oystercatchers were to me. A catalyst propelling her on to a new path.

But why, you may ask, do curlews need help? And why should you, reading this, care, when there are people like Mary and Curlew Action fighting for them? Curlews nest on farmland and in upland areas and it's here they are facing a couple of issues. First, the intensification of farming to keep up with feeding a growing population of us humans means that we have changed the way we farm and, in turn, destroyed their nesting sites. With climate change, we are seeing more flooding, which is again destroying these areas. The UK has the densest population of foxes in Europe, with them and other predators thriving as a result of our throwaway society, and these predators feed on, yes, you guessed it, ground nesting birds. And then there's upland forestry, which brings yet more issues for the curlew. With an increase in planting, trees are being placed on their nesting sites, removing the available spaces for them to raise their chicks. Whichever issue you focus on, it seems apparent that our actions are essentially stopping curlews at the source, preventing them from continuing the lines, and an estimated 10,000 chicks per year are just not being 'produced'. That's a ridiculously high number in a single species. The UK has lost an estimated 65 per cent of breeding birds since 1970. When Mary realised this, she also recognised that we don't have long to do something to change this.

I asked Mary why she does what she does, how she gets up every day to fight again for her beloved curlews, and she told me the one piece of advice that her editor gave her when she was writing her stunning book, *Curlew Moon*. They told her when she felt lost, and didn't know which direction to turn, to 'go back to the birds'. This seems like good advice, and I know that I should do the same.

Mary doesn't call herself 'a birder'. Like me, she came to realise there was a whole world populated by lives that continue on despite us humans. 'If I'm ever feeling claustrophobic in the human world, I remember what my editor told me,' she tells me. 'There's so much more in this world to focus on than just the people in it and, in fact, the world seems better when you realise that.'

Since starting Curlew Action, Mary's words and work have had a great impact in helping educate people about curlews and that's because of her determination to put herself out there and just do whatever she can. Her mission also has royal support. In 2018, then Prince Charles (now King Charles), who apparently loves a curlew, organised two symposiums about them. This is good but what happens to the birds who don't have royal backing? Who speaks for them? People like Mary. And, if you think about it, if you're passionate enough about it, that could be me or you. What are you passionate about and how far would you go to protect it?

As part of Curlew Action, Mary initiated 'World Curlew Day' on 21 April 2017, an opportunity for the world to celebrate a bird that really needs our help and to get people talking about it. It's largely a reason I felt I wanted to include them in this book; the curlews really deserve some big public love. Mary chose that date as it's also the Festival of St Beuno, the patron saint of curlews. Beuno was a seventh-century Welsh abbot; the legend goes that he dropped his book of sermons into the sea where it disappeared from view. The book reappeared on a stone, a safe distance from the tide, with a curlew guarding it after having picked it up and moved it to safety. Beuno was so overwhelmed with gratitude that he prayed for protection for the bird and that, so they say, is why it's so challenging to locate curlew nests. While you may not be able to spy curlews every day, you can spread the joy, talk about them, share information with friends who may then, in turn, share that with more people, snowballing until every one of us is aware of the plight of this enchantingly brilliant bird.

As if fighting for curlews isn't enough, Mary has realised the importance of grasping that wonder in nature we all have as children. That's why Mary has been campaigning for a GCSE in natural history to be added to the national curriculum. She began her petition in 2011, when it was initially shot down by the government, which claimed it was already covered in the curriculum. (I must have missed that lesson in school.) To gain extra support, Mary launched a government petition in 2017. A pivotal turn of events occurred when the former Green Party MP Caroline Lucas offered her support to it, along with Tim Oates, Director of Research and Development for Cambridge Assessment, an education department of Cambridge University. Running consultation during the pandemic, the team wrote the specification, which was accepted in 2022, but unfortunately at the time of writing, it has not been finalised and the battle to get a Natural History GCSE in schools goes on.

I'm trying to imagine how different my journey might have been if there was a natural history GCSE when I did my exams. Admittedly, I only did the final year of GCSEs, moving back from France halfway through that period and scraping through with an A in French and average grades in everything else (except maths, which we won't mention). Had it been available, would I have chosen it as one of my options? Was it too late for me by then, my imagination far from birds, captured by dreams of being a West End musical star? If I'd been tuned into the right frequency at fifteen instead of in my late twenties, would I have found that my passions lay elsewhere? Or was it just not the right time for me then? While it is absolutely incredible that there may soon be a natural history option available to my own children if they so wish, by fifteen has that wonder we had when we were young already started to fade?

The focus on nature needs to start much, much earlier, in my opinion, during a child's educational journey, capturing that natural curiosity children have. Otherwise, unless kids have parents who take them out on journeys to share the natural spectacles and things they love, who cry over the arrival of a swift during the summer, and encourage them to get down in the dirt to identify bugs on every walk, teenagers just won't be inclined to take the GCSE. We need to make nature 'cool' (which it obviously is, I mean, have you seen it?!). Otherwise the only kids who will choose the GCSE are those who have had the guiding hand of nature nerd parents or other influential people in their lives and the echo chamber will continue. If you have a child then, please, encourage their wonder, even if sometimes you feel like you don't have time to answer yet another question or look at yet another leaf or twig. Slow down. Indulge them. Embrace curiosity. Not just theirs, but yours too.

I asked Mary for some final words of advice for those who are perhaps at the beginning of their journey into nature, or in fact any stage of the adventure. 'My advice is to pick something to love and love it. Love it with everything you have. Through the ups and downs, the sugar-pink bits as well as the bad times. Love is powerful but not easy, we all know that, but we won't save something unless we love it.'

Find love, and hold on to it. It sounds obvious, doesn't it, but I often feel this world could do with a lot less doom and gloom, and a never-ending stream of love. I think we all could do with that!

Despite our efforts to make nature cool and accepted in mainstream society, and the amount of people from all walks of life who are popping up on social media, on TV and streaming services, in books, on podcasts, sharing their passion for the natural world and doing their best to share the love, I keep hearing stories about people being bullied as kids for their passion. With toxicity such a topic of discussion, why are we still raising kids who feel it's okay to belittle someone for their interests? I can't even fathom that mindset.

Someone who experienced this as a child but who came through the other side, without letting go of that love, is Sarah Cunningham. Sarah is a friend, community engagement officer for the Birda app, and part of a women's birders group chat that I'm part of on WhatsApp. To be honest, I linger on the edges of the group chat while they discuss the birds they have seen and want to see, offering up the occasional pigeon or blurred photo of a bird for them to ID for me, which they always willingly do.

Sarah told me that, like a lot of people, her love for birds began in the garden with an RSPB children's magazine and a bird book which she carried everywhere, even in her school bag. Unfortunately, in an all too familiar story, Sarah was bullied for her interests and encountered kids who would mock her, ripping pages out from her birding books (again, who is teaching these kids that this is okay?). Luckily, Sarah didn't let this deter her. Her parents actively encouraged her, taking her on visits to nature reserves and helping her to join local wildlife groups. Sarah told me that nature is where she feels safest, a place of comfort. It rings true and is an echo of what so many of the people I've spoken to feel, myself included.

'Nature was, and still is, a constant mood regulator. Growing up, nobody my age really understood my love for nature and birds. I had some amazing teachers who saw my interests and enhanced them. My family was also a great support. So many happy memories are of walking around nature reserves, trying to spot kingfishers and ospreys. Nature has been the foundation for so many powerful friendships in my life. Sharing that common love for birds and the outdoors instantly makes you feel you know someone already. Nature is how I have had the most interesting conversations with strangers, met incredible life-changing friends and is also how I met my life-long partner. Who knew watching puffins together on a seabird colony could spark love?'

Sarah is the living embodiment of everything I want to communicate in this book. She's someone who loves and lives her passion for nature, a positive ray of sunshine who brings silly magical fun to situations. A birding trip with Sarah is a great adventure where she fills the space with her pure joy. To be quite honest, I wish I could capture her feelings and experience of the natural world, bottle it, reproduce it and give it to everyone so that we all might revel in a small slice of that wonder. It's that feeling we need to find a way to spread and share, and as I can't bottle it, the best I can do is share these stories in the hope that you, too, will find a way to the magic in the everyday.

I've got a bright green, metal water bottle from Mountain Warehouse that bears the message, 'never lose your sense of wonder'. I used to mock this message, comparing it to a 'live, laugh, love' plaque hanging in someone's downstairs loo, but the more I think about it, the more I agree with the sentiment, and that's the message, the lesson, of this chapter, and what I wish for my children. *Never* lose your sense of wonder. If we can figure out a way to cling on to that, own it and make it a default setting in our lives, I think the world would suddenly seem better, be better. As I finish typing that sentence, a small, female house sparrow lands in my window feeder, knocking against the window as she picks through the birdseed to find the bit she wants. My mind wanders for a second, wondering, which seed does she want? Where is she flying back to? Who is she? Now my eyes are open again, I don't think I'll ever stop wondering.

Nor do I want to.

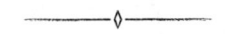

---◊---

Picture a bird about the size of a starling with a sleek, silky plumage that shimmers in the sunlight. Upon closer inspection, the waxwing's beauty truly comes to light. Its soft, cinnamon feathers are complemented by a delicate smudge of pale yellow on its belly. The wings are adorned with a splash of vibrant red on the secondary feathers and a small patch of brilliant white at the tips, resembling drops of melted wax, which is, I can only assume, how it got its name. The waxwing's most distinctive feature is perhaps its sleek crest that it can raise or lower at will, adding an air of elegance, a certain *je ne sais quoi* to its appearance. It has a black mask extending from the base of its beak to its piercing eyes, giving it a mysterious, almost sneaky expression. In the winter months, waxwings are known to migrate to the UK in search of food, often forming large flocks that descend upon red berry trees which they hoover up effortlessly. Their arrival is a spectacle that attracts birders, photographers and general nature lovers as the trees come alive.

Obviously, I'd never heard of a waxwing, let alone seen one, before my epiphany. Once I became aware of their existence, seeing one became a bit of an obsession, which resulted in two fruitless winters where I somehow managed to miss every single sighting. Every time I received a text from friends in the area declaring, 'Waxwings in Sheringham, come and see them,' I'd race down only to find I was too late, and they had vanished. It's only January but I have to say 2024 is beginning to look like it'll be no different.

'Waxwings in Wiveton by the church,' a text from Chris Stone pings through once again.

*Is there even any point in me trying?* I wonder.

I'm halfway through a really long Teams meeting that could have been a Post-it note, so I make the decision to pop down before the school run and see if, on the off chance, I can spot one. I pull up to the place where I know they have been seen and, of course, there is literally no one here. If there was a waxwing here, this area would be filled with photographers and scopes all scrambling to catch a glimpse of these beautiful birds. I don't even bother getting out of the car, admitting defeat, once again assuming that this is another winter where I won't be seeing a waxwing.

'Waxwings are there again today,' Chris texts temptingly the next day and I am torn – do I bother? It's only five minutes down the road but I know how this is going to go. Yet, not one to give up easily, I get in the car and decide to give it a try.

I pull up in a small car park in Wiveton, a village in North Norfolk not far from the coast, and immediately my hope soars when I spot around twenty people standing with scopes pointing towards some tall trees which are covered in bright red berries. I open the boot of the car, then mutter, 'Shit, the scope is in the conservatory.'

And once again kick myself for my failure to plan ahead. My phone has got a good zoom, so that'll have to do. I spot a couple sharing a scope, on a path set back from the crowd taking turns to look down the lens.

'Have you seen the waxwings?' I ask, approaching them.

'Yes!' the woman replies excitedly and kindly lets me have a look through their scope. Sure enough, five shiny birds are hanging in all directions on a series of branches, looking like the front of a Christmas card as they nip at the berries.

Sue and John, the couple with the scope, tell me they are new to birding and still trying to work out what everything is. *Me, too,* I think but don't say out loud. And we stand together and share in the moment, chatting about the birds and how amazing it is that we have the opportunity to see them. I am still in a state of disbelief that I have finally managed to catch up with this elusive (to me at least) species.

I leave the site elated and feeling full of joy, and my phone buzzes in my pocket. It's Luke, a local friend and owner of a fitness studio in the town. 'Why are there a load of people with binoculars and big lens cameras outside my house?' the text reads. 'Dunno, I'll come round and see,' I reply, curious at what it could possibly be. Luke lives on a quiet street, surrounded on all sides by houses and a large private school that dominates the centre of the town.

'Waxwings on that rowan tree,' a man with a camera says cheerily as I arrive, pointing to the large tree that sits at the end of Luke's drive. Luke, who is standing at the end of his drive with his arms folded, looks at the crowd gathered and laughs at my excitement when I move next to him to tell him what all the fuss is about. 'I've heard of them but didn't expect them in the middle of the town, especially on my drive.' Luke has a general appreciation of nature, but still laughs at me when we are in a PT session and I stop mid-squat to take a video of a caterpillar or to look at a swift sailing past.

'Neither did I,' I reply as I stare at these beautiful birds.

It seems waxwings are like buses: you wait for ages, then two come along at once.

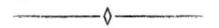

---◊---

It's February 2024 and I pull into a narrow-gated entrance. I lean out of the car window to type in the code to the silver pin pad. The tall, green metal gate swings open, and as I drive forward, I see Matt Spracklen, a.k.a. the Rock 'n' Roll Birder, standing by his car wearing a light brown suede coat, skinny jeans and black pointed boots. His dark hair and perfectly styled beard frame the aviator sunglasses that are pushed against his face, despite the drizzle that is threatening. He certainly stands out on a nature reserve, and to be quite honest it's refreshing to see someone who looks so unique, standing there confidently with his binoculars, ready for a walk around Kempton Nature Reserve, a members-only reserve built on a decommissioned Thames Water reservoir. It stands as a little natural oasis not far from Hampton Court, a constant stream of planes from nearby Heathrow passing over the top, as countless species seem to coexist with these metal birds.

Matt doesn't work in conservation or in the nature industry. In fact, away from his Instagram persona and recently launched Rock 'n Roll Birder podcast, he is a country music radio presenter and a musician. For a long time, he tells me, he didn't have time to look at birds. He was always into nature; in fact, as a kid he was often late for school as he was looking at birds or reading his birding books. This feels reminiscent of my own experience with my children, running late because we have seen the first swift of the year, which feels more pressing than being on time for registration.

# CURLEW

Matt tells me that his teacher attributed his learning to read to his bird books. Despite being a bird nerd since birth, Matt feels he isn't an expert and embraces the fact that he is always presented with opportunities to learn, and I love that about him: he's not afraid to admit when he doesn't know something, it doesn't matter. What is apparent and inspiring is his willingness and readiness to learn.

We sit down in the first hide, and for a moment we're in silence as a chorus of strange sounds come from the pool in front of us. The only way I can think to describe it is the opening of that Disturbed song, 'Down with the Sickness' (quickly Google it if you don't know). Yeah. That's the sound coming from the water. Definitely not a bird. Matt gets his binoculars on the water (mine are in the car), and we discover that it's in fact a group of toads chilling in the shallows. Who knew that toads are into Nu Metal?

We sit in the hide for what seems like hours, chatting and looking out of the window. Matt tells me that he has been lucky enough to work and play music in the most brilliant places. He studied country music in Nashville, played in a punk band for a while, but in 2020 during lockdown he had his birding revival. It started with trying to bring birds to the garden with feeders and seeing what he could see. Soon, curiosity became an obsession, and he found himself living the double life of a musician and birder. Perhaps the most interesting revelation from Matt is that he is colour blind.

'Does that cause any issues when you're looking at birds?' I ask, wondering what the parakeets, streaks of lime screeching across the sky, must look like without that trademark green plumage.

## THE LIFE-AFFIRMING MAGIC OF BIRDS

'ID can be a problem,' he responds honestly, 'but I'm learning to rely on other senses to know what birds are. It's like a different type of awareness, forcing me to connect with the environment on a deeper level.' Suddenly I'm a bit envious of Matt and the way he must experience the world, and I immediately decide to start actively applying my other senses to heighten my own experience.

The door of the hide opens and two older gentlemen clatter in with cameras and binoculars. 'Ooh, people,' one of the men, with something Bernard Cribbins-esque about him, announces in a south London accent.

'That's you frightened off then, Col,' the other mocks.

The men settle themselves in and we soon fall into conversation. Colin and Franko, as they introduce themselves, have both been regular visitors to the site for over thirty years and have seen the changes in the landscape and species. Now they are retired, they pop down every day for a look and a leg stretch.

'Why every day?' I ask, curious to know what brings them here.

'To be honest, my wife can't get out anymore. I have a terminally ill son and I need something to hold on to.' Colin surprises me with his blunt honesty. To hear someone, a man, of his generation admit that he spends time in nature for his mental health is refreshing, and as the conversation continues, he tells us that he wishes young people would pay more attention to the older generation.

'We've been there, we understand how things work and want to pass on that information so you lot can enjoy all this,' he gestures at the water outside, which is reflecting the trees and a British Airways plane that is taking off full of holidaymakers.

'That's fair,' Matt muses, 'but equally, younger people want to be heard, too. A lot of us are passionate about all this,' gesturing at the same scene, 'and embrace that it's changing.'

'Perhaps,' says Franko, 'we should all try listening to each other, especially you, Col.' Colin shoots Franko a mock stern look. 'He's one of them climate change deniers,' adds Franko, chuckling.

'Nah, Franko, I'm one of them realistic buggers who looks at facts,' Colin replies. The two of them fall into a light-hearted bicker as we edge out of the hide, bidding them a good day, as we carry on our day with the realisation that, whoever we are, whatever we believe to be true, wherever we come from, nature is there for us. If we choose to let it be.

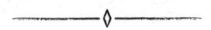

———◊———

Wollaton Hall is a Grade I-listed Elizabethan manor house that feels as though it has been misplaced in the middle of Nottingham. Like someone has put it down on the way to the rolling countryside of the Peak District, just an hour away, and forgot to pick it up again.

Pulling off the busy main road in the car on this day in March 2024, the atmosphere changes from a harsh city vibe to a quiet suburban, tree-lined street and eventually, if you keep going, you turn through two large, black wooden gates that welcome you into the parkland. You pass a mural painted on the café next to a packed play area, where images of mice, flowers and bees welcome you out of the city and into a rolling green space.

I drive past a tree-lined avenue and look to my left and get a glimpse of the hall, which was used as Batman's house in the latest incarnations of the masked crusader films, and spot two Egyptian geese swaying across the path, bringing the scene to life.

Getting out of the car I spot a ranger I know here who spends much of his time volunteering in Africa with rhinos, and shout across the car park, 'Johnny! Have you seen Kyle?' I'm here today to meet with Kyle Heesom, who is a ranger with an unexpected journey into nature that I'm keen to hear about.

Johnny points me in the direction of where the lesser-spotted Kyle was last seen, and I stick my brightly coloured wellies on and squelch my way across the fields, away from the Elizabethan manor, whose walls call out to me with stories of Tudor residents and a vast history.

There are a lot of dog walkers out this morning, and looking around I spot a figure in a black waterproof and beanie hat, appearing to be in heated debate with a couple who have two labradors bounding around them, getting unnervingly close to a herd of red deer lying peacefully in the long grass.

'Hi, Kyle.' I greet him as he walks away from the couple, who move on, dogs still running freely off the lead.

'They'll be the first to kick off when that stag goes for the dog.' His broad Nottingham accent is filled with irritation from a conversation he has to have all too often with visitors to the parkland that he manages. Kyle has always been big into nature, a fact he attributes to his dad, who was a keen fisherman and birdwatcher. His journey into nature hasn't been an easy one, though. As we walk across the muddy field, he tells me that nature has felt like a guilty pleasure, or a taboo subject, when it really shouldn't be.

'Being a typical lad from Bulwell, football, girls and nature didn't really fit together,' he explains. 'No one around me was even remotely interested in nature so I kept it quiet. This one lad in high school used to try and bully me, calling me a "nature nerd".'

'Oh,' I reply, 'I think nature nerd is a cool title.'

'Yeah, so do I now, proudly wear that badge.'

We come to the edge of the large lake where the image of the manor house is reflected perfectly in the water. The image ripples as a Canada goose glides past.

'There's a heron that nests on that island every year.' Kyle gestures towards a small lump of land in the middle of the lake.

As a child and teenager, Kyle would spend every spring looking for bird nests and ticking them off a list in his head. He recounts a memory of finding a bullfinch nest, the bright male looking back at him through the hedgerow as he peered in. He never disturbed the nests, but just spent time looking, observing, falling in love over and over again with the species within.

'It felt like a balancing act for ages. I felt like I lived two lives at one point. It was like being a tracksuit-wearing, slang-talking chav and being passionate about nature didn't work together. No matter what I did, I felt out of place. So, depending on who I was with or what I was doing, I had to hide the other side of me and I had to adjust my personality to the person or the situation I was in at that time,' Kyle says with a hint of regret.

'What would you tell your younger self?' I ask.

'If I could give advice to my younger self, it would be "be yourself! Your people will come to you!"' It's decent advice that we could all do with listening to.

## THE LIFE-AFFIRMING MAGIC OF BIRDS

The lake is alive with birds, the air filled with voices of families who are visiting the park, grabbing a drink from the coffee van whose generator buzzes in the background.

'I remember when I was at Brackenhurst College doing my Countryside Management diploma, it felt like the lecturers looked at me and didn't take me seriously. I remember seeing the first swallow of the year and no one else noticed. The lecturer laughed at me and said, "It was probably a pigeon." Doubting me as if I was not capable of identifying a swallow! Why did he assume I was wrong in the first place? Was it the way I looked or spoke?'

I put my leg on a log and roll it back gently to unveil a family of woodlice which immediately scatter in the unexpected sunlight. 'So, if there was such an internal battle going on between how the world saw you and who you wanted to be, what made you suddenly decide to jump to where you are now?' I'm genuinely curious to know how Kyle went from hiding his passion for the natural world, to being a manager of a glorious parkland.

'My "butterfly effect" moment was getting sacked from B&M at nineteen years old for texting in sick. I think as I got older, I just gave less of a shit what people thought. Now I talk about nature and publish it online. I do still get the odd comment, but I don't give it the time of day now.'

I love that Kyle eventually just went for it. Now, he regularly fights with councils when he sees them cutting back hedgerows in nesting season, and recently won a battle to stop the council mowing wildflower verges during the summer.

'Do you think it's changing? Is nature cool yet?' I wonder out loud.

'Attitudes are changing, slowly. People with a variety of backgrounds are showcasing their love for nature online,' he tells me, 'and in the media, which can only have a positive effect on people watching it who live in urban areas with limited green spaces.'

I roll the log back into place, putting the roof back on the woodlice house, and a woodpecker drums in the distance. Kyle and I smile at each other as we silently acknowledge the sound which goes unnoticed by the people around us. 'Being a nature nerd is the new cool I reckon,' Kyle goes on. 'I'm not worried about admitting it, oh, and I still wear a tracksuit and talk like a chav from Bulwell, innit.' He laughs.

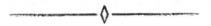

---

The cold air pierces through the layers of my fleece and thick coat as I step out of the car and into the misty embrace of the early morning. Sleep eluded me this morning, so I decided I'd had enough of tossing and turning, and I sought solace in the solitude of the coast. Nothing worse than being alone in a house and unable to sleep, thoughts swirling in my head. The kids are spending the weekend at their dad's, my mum is in Liverpool with my grandma and so it's just me this weekend.

I've never been very good at being alone, but somehow being outside in nature right now makes me feel like there's more to this existence than a brief moment of anxiety-induced insomnia. The faint glow of first light dances on the horizon, casting a pale hue over the North Norfolk landscape. The air is heavy with that scent of salt from the shingle beach that I know to be somewhere at the end of this path, and the sound of crashing waves echoes in the distance.

## THE LIFE-AFFIRMING MAGIC OF BIRDS

As I walk along the rugged track, large stones have been churned up by last night's rain and I move between them and the patches of mud. It's oddly silent. Even the wintery birds aren't awake yet. A shadow of a large hare darts across the path ahead of me, the first suggestion of a life that isn't mine this morning. The quiet is broken by a haunting cry that moves like a ghost somewhere beyond my vision. I'm still rubbish at bird sounds; there are only a few that I can identify with any certainty and this is one of them. It's the unmistakable call of a curlew, its mournful song sending shivers down my spine. The sound envelops me in its strange melody. I stop, feeling both elated and melancholic as the sound grows louder, shouting out across the fields.

The curlew's call, as a musician once said to Mary Colwell, is an interesting combination of major and minor keys due to the structure of the bird's syrinx. This weird blend evokes a mixture of emotions within me every time I hear it. There's a sense of happiness in its lilting notes, like a cheery song on the radio on a Sunday morning, but it's tinged with an underlying uncertainty, like a shadow lurking in the depths of the melody. It's as if the bird itself is caught between worlds, its song a reflection of the liminal space between its own survival and the impact that humans are having on the species. A call that speaks of delighted ancestral memories, and concern and heartbreak for the future.

I strain my ears, trying to pinpoint the source of the sound, but a thin wintery mist obscures my vision, shrouding me in a haze. I know the curlew is out there somewhere, hidden from view but right there in its ethereal song. Somewhere in the fields that flank my path, there will be one, maybe more, waiting, wondering, hoping.

As light breaks through the clouds, illuminating me with shades of pink and blue in a way only the North Norfolk coast knows how, I feel that familiar sense of peace wash over me, the feeling that nature brings when it knows I need it the most. The curlew's song fades into the background, but its echoes linger in my mind, a reminder of the magic that lies just beyond my veil of reality. As I walk on towards the sound of the waves to dip my toes in the freezing sea and awaken my soul in the physical sense, the world around me begins to wake up, coming to life. The birdsongs blend into each other and I am unable to pick out any individual sounds, yet the curlew song sings on in my memory. The soundtrack to the wonder that I hope will never fade.

# 9
# GOOSE

*'One touch of nature makes the whole world kin.'*
*– Troilus and Cressida*, Act 3, Scene 3

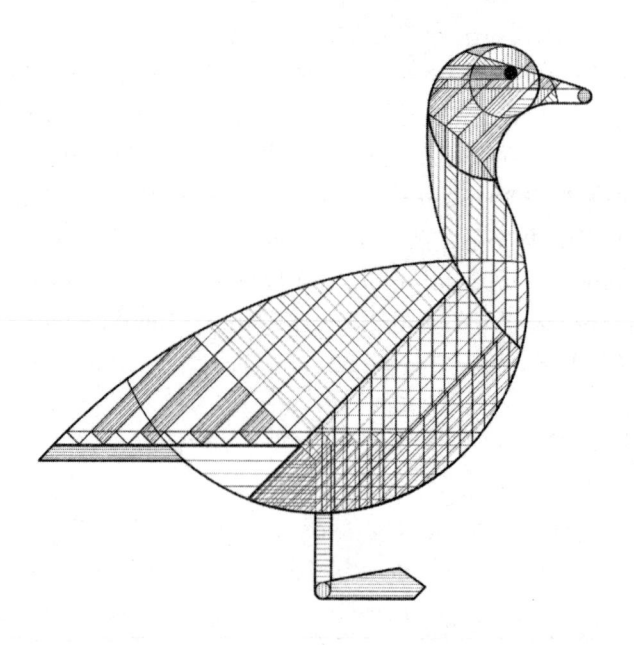

**The world can be so much bigger when you let nature in**

My relationship with geese hasn't always been a positive one. In fact, I'd say I used to have quite negative feelings towards geese. And by geese, I mean the ones you find around ponds and sitting confidently in busy public parks, hissing at unsuspecting passers-by. Like me.

Thoses are usually greylags, grey geese with a bright orange beak, and Canada geese, tall birds with sleek black heads and necks. I'd never heard of a pink-footed goose, had no idea there were species that travel thousands of miles each year to join us here in the UK from their Arctic breeding grounds. I spent most of my life unaware of the incredible journeys taking place throughout the year made by these birds or that there were nine unique species of geese which can be seen around the UK. If you'd asked me to tell you about a Taiga bean goose, I would have suggested you were making it up. In fact, I'd hazard a guess that a lot of you out there hold some negative feelings towards geese, possibly based on an encounter with them in a park or wood. Ask someone to imagine a goose and I bet the image they'll conjure up will be one of a big, white, hissing farm goose and, yes, my first thoughts were exactly that for a long time. In fact, I'll admit I was a bit scared of geese. Silly really. The world is a beautiful place if you let yourself see.

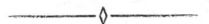

———◊———

In September 2018, I made the decision to take back control of my life and do something positive for me. After a couple of years of my identity being purely 'Mummy', I knew it was time to find myself again – or possibly for the first time. The past has always fascinated me. I think it stems from a fortunate childhood filled with trips to National Trust properties and museums. Holidays weren't sitting on the beach and relaxing; they were stomping around ancient Greek ruins and exploring the most bizarre rural locations in the US in pursuit of knowledge. My last holiday with my dad before I fell pregnant with my first child, just a few months later, was a week-long tour of the beaches of Normandy, exploring every corner of the D-Day museums and marvelling at the Bayeux Tapestry. How many people give 'archaeologist' as their answer when you ask them what they wanted to be as a kid? Well, I did. I decided to take that childhood dream and, at twenty-five-years old, go and get a degree in the subject.

Over the three years spent at the University of York, my eyes were opened to subjects I'd never even thought about. I started the degree with an obsession with the Tudors and Stuarts, an obsession I still have, and left with a dissertation about the last common ancestor between humans, chimpanzees and bonobos. I had no idea the subject of archaeology was so vast and yet here I was, exploring every inch of it. This may sound like just another impulsive jump to add to the list. Much like doing a degree as a mature student, or moving to Wales with my children in pursuit of the next chapter of my journey. But my leap from one subject to another is, to me at least, testament to the eye-opening, life-changing experience that my degree was.

As soon as I stepped through the doors to that university, opportunities were presented to me that I never knew existed, let alone thought were possible for me. Whoever commented that your uni years are the best years of your life, wasn't lying. Only mine weren't filled with the standard uni experiences that I saw in my cohort, the newfound freedom of being eighteen and away from parental bounds. Instead, mine was a juggling act between all the different parts of my life. Parenting, working, studying, trying to find time to come up for air in the desperate quest to complete the course and achieve something with my life. All of these aspects weighed down upon me, and I hadn't yet realised that there was something waiting on my doorstep that would become a form of free therapy for me. Nature was waiting to help me, it was literally right there – I just couldn't see it yet.

Sometimes, one of the children would have to accompany me to lectures and seminars if they weren't at nursery; sometimes I would type out an email to my supervisor, Dr Nathan Wales, declaring that it was all too much and I was withdrawing from the degree. But somehow, with the help of my mum and the most supportive group of friends – Lu, Bryony, Giselle, all either parents or 'mature students' also juggling in their own personal circuses – we all did it together. We made it out of there with that all important piece of paper that says, 'you've done it, you're not lazy, you don't lack dedication'. All of the phrases that had been thrown at me during my schooldays were null and void. I'd achieved a degree.

———◊———

The main campus of the University of York is split into two main parts, East Campus and West Campus. Both are unsuspecting nature havens hidden among towering teaching blocks and 1960s student accommodation, brown brick walls giving it a somewhat oppressive feel, particularly on a gloomy day like today. It's October 2018 and I'm walking through a corridor of concrete, my footsteps echoing on the empty, grey stone path. The only human sound is the bumping of my bag as it bounces against my back as I walk. It's strange to see the campus so empty. I imagine the buildings around me, the first-year accommodation block filled with nervous new students, fresh out of school and plunged into an independent living situation for the first time in their lives. Pizza boxes and empty bottles of vodka line the windowsills of most of the kitchens I can see into. A cardboard cutout of Danny DeVito stares at me from a third-floor window.

I'm heading to the YEAR Centre, the York Experimental Archaeology Research Centre, a brilliant plot of land that hides behind an imposing building which houses the environmental and biological studies. The YEAR centre is a dream for any archaeology student, with a Mesolithic hut recreated in one corner, a Viking forge and a central firepit where experts will teach you how to knap flint into wonky stone axe-heads. As I said, I found myself doing a lot of things on that degree that I could never have imagined.

I'm walking along the edge of the campus lake now. A body of murky water stretches for almost a mile across the campus where the landscape changes from crumbling concrete building blocks and brand new, all singing and dancing departments, to sweeping lawns, ornate gardens and weeping willows that touch the surface of the water as you head towards Heslington Hall. This Victorian Jacobean-style manor house now forms part of the administration department and hosts dinners and networking sessions for academics at the university. Now, if there's one thing that York Uni is famous for, and what former students will unite over, it's the geese.

Ask anyone who has had anything to do with York Uni and they will be able to tell you a story about the geese. The geese are well known for chasing down students on their way to lectures, hissing as they approach and encouraging people to walk 'the long way round' rather than face the daunting prospect of walking through a gaggle of them. I'd be very rich if I had a pound for every group of students I've seen stop, consider their next move and divert to avoid these seemingly aggressive birds. I'm one of those students who will cut through buildings to avoid confrontation, and as I walk in the direction of my destination, five Canada geese are settled right in the middle of the path. I only know they are Canada geese because of an old, dirt covered information board which tells passers-by about the wildlife living on the lake. The dust layer across it tells me it is largely ignored.

Ten eyes whip round and stare at me as I approach. One of the geese stands up and walks towards me, hissing, with its head down as it draws closer. I have no choice but to carry on. I'm running slightly behind schedule and don't have time to let a group of birds disrupt my day. So, slightly anxiously and taking care to not make eye contact with the aggressor and its gang, I tiptoe through the group, ignoring the fact that all heads turn to watch me as I move away swiftly. A safe distance away, I spot Long Boi walking along the edge of the lake through a muddy patch of grass.

Long Boi was a university, and now national, celebrity. He was an Indian Runner duck, a species of duck which stand almost upright and look like small, feathered humans next to the more 'ordinary' ducks you may be used to seeing at your local pond. Little is known about how Long Boi came to be a resident at the university, perhaps as an unwanted pet, but over time students, who preferred this gentle natured duck to the angry geese, fed him and helped him settle. Long Boi shot to fame when, for some reason, James Corden mentioned him on his *Late Late Show* in 2021. Footballer Peter Crouch shared a tweet about the duck saying 'that's my kind of duck'. Then Greg James, Radio One DJ, who took a shine to Long Boi, featured him on his breakfast show where he quacked for the nation. Sadly though, in May 2023, the university put out a statement (this is how loved Long Boi was by the university community) saying he hadn't been seen for a few months and was presumed dead.

This is well before that time, and I bend down to snap a quick photo of the campus celebrity but let out a yelp of surprise and leap forward as I feel something pinch my leg. Turning, I see the figure of the Canada goose hurry away from me. It's bitten the back of my calf, through my jeans, to let me know I'm still not welcome.

Humans are, by default, storytellers. For millennia, telling stories has been a way of sharing experience and information, to entertain and to inform. But it strikes me that our reality is shaped by the stories that we happen to encounter. Of course, if we find ourselves in an echo chamber full of people who have heard the same stories as us, then that becomes the norm and we find ourselves stuck, unable to move on from that reality until someone else enlightens us with a retelling. I suppose that's how it was for me with geese, and with herring gulls, too. I'd been told repeatedly that geese weren't our friends, they're aggressive, they'll bite. (Well, true, in my experience.) Gulls will attack you, be careful, don't leave food out, otherwise they'll grab it. The classic – 'swans will break your arm'.

Once I opened up to a different narrative and started to listen to other versions of the story, I started to see all of these species in a different light. Geese, no matter the species, are extremely protective, both of their nests and of their personal space. Me, too. The species that tend to live around humans, unfortunately, have given themselves a bad name by displaying these traits and being dubbed as aggressive, when in fact, like all of us, they're just doing what they can to survive. So, despite their sometimes spiky exterior, the geese you encounter are just fighting to secure their space in this chaotic world we have created. What people don't see is that underneath the feathers and attitude are incredibly tight bonds between family groups. Geese, along with cranes and swans, are among the only birds which will take on epic migration journeys with their family groups. Often, birds will tackle these journeys alone, travelling thousands of miles through treacherous conditions on solo flights. In some species, the parents will migrate before their young, flying off to warmer climes without so much as a backwards glance, as the juveniles check in for their first long haul flight. Knowing this gave me a new affection for geese. Now, when I see the skeins of geese flying above me every day in autumn, I think of all the families up there making the trip together, leaving no one behind. Geese have a lot to teach us about working together.

When you see geese flying in formation, they're actually working together to make the trip a little bit easier for everyone, their flapping wings creating lift to carry their group members. If a goose is tired or unwell and falls behind, two other geese will fall back with it and support it until it is ready to rejoin the flock, where they will work together to catch up. When flying long distances, they will keep changing the leader of the pack so that no one goose has to take full responsibility and become overly exhausted.

'GEESE!' Jack screams from the conservatory as his brother and I rush to his side to see if he's winding us up. It's October 2023 and I can hear the calls of the birds quickly approaching, and grabbing the key to the French doors, I open them and release Jack into the garden. He stands on the garden table, presumably to get a better vantage point, and waits. No more than thirty seconds later, they come into view. Hundreds of shapes in a V-formation pass over our heads, in the direction of their feeding grounds for the first time this season, filling the sky with honking calls. The creators of this glorious sound? Pink-footed geese. Now this is what autumn is all about.

―――◊―――

Pink-footed geese are a species which spend their summers in the Arctic, before flying to the UK in the autumn to spend their winter feasting on sugar beet crops and grass. For me, since moving to Norfolk, they have become a symbol of the season, which doesn't really start until the air is filled with the calls as thousands of individuals storm across the big coastal skies.

Just like if you'd asked me a few years ago about a Taiga bean goose, I would have suggested you were making it up if you'd told me that I would be spending a Saturday evening on a chilly Norfolk beach, waiting to see my first pink-footed geese of the season. I would have laughed. They say that birding sneaks up on you, and as I walk along the boardwalk through the tall pine trees at Holkham in pursuit of a bird experience, I realise the truth in that statement.

# GOOSE

The pink-footed geese are one of the great nature spectacles of the Norfolk coast, their loud calls providing the soundtrack to autumn mornings and evenings as they fly over in large skeins in search for freshly harvested sugar beet left over by busy farmers as they gather up their crops. Everyone locally seems to have seen or at least heard the geese already, fresh reports of them popping up on my social media feeds every time I refresh the phone screen. Autumn is closing in, summer a distant memory as we hurtle towards the colder months. I need to experience this spectacle to lift me out of a sad funk I seem to have found myself stuck in recently. *How can that cheer you up? They're just geese*, you may be thinking. I would have thought that too if I hadn't had a Christmas goose encounter a few years ago. Admittedly that sounds a bit like the ending of *A Christmas Carol*. I think it's a goose that Ebeneezer Scrooge nearly purchases for Bob Cratchit's family at the end of the Dickens classic, before deciding on the more exotic and extravagant turkey. Thankfully, no ghosts of Christmas past visited me when I sat alone in my campervan on Christmas Day in 2023. Perhaps if they had, they could have kept me company, as I spent the first Christmas Day of my entire life alone.

My children were at their dad's house and the rest of my family too far away to make the journey for the sake of one day. I never realised how Christmas made me feel. I'd always cast it aside as 'just a day', enjoying the lead-up to Christmas and seeing the boys' faces when they came downstairs on the big day. But sitting alone in my rusty Transit camper (which I had to scrap a few months later when the floor fell out – yes, literally), I realise that the magic of Christmas is about being together. I felt a crushing sense of loneliness that I'd never felt before.

I sat on the step of the van looking out on to an empty campsite. The owner had left the dinner table with his family to welcome me; I could feel the pity in his demeanour as he directed me towards the deserted field. But still, it felt better than sitting on my own in the house watching re-runs of Christmas TV specials with a roast dinner for one. As I waited for the water to boil very slowly on my tiny gas stove so I could make a cup of peppermint tea before bed, I zipped my fleece up fully to try and counter the chilly wind that was building with a threatening storm coming in from the sea.

The sun had almost set, but the sky was still illuminated and above me was a screen of deep indigo, the absolute epitome of a twilight sky. A few black outlines of clouds wisped along the scene, breaking up the colour with hints of the darkness that was about to descend, a metaphor for my mood. The sky was still and the only sound I could hear apart from the distant waves was the hissing gas flame coming from my stove, desperately trying to heat up the water that stood, lukewarm still, in the kettle above.

A sound stood out against the stillness, an unmistakable chorus of honks and cackles drawing closer and closer. As I stood up and moved so I could see past the van, a billow of pink-footed geese streamed towards me on their way to their roosting site. Thousands of outlines above me, just visible against the navy blue sky. I stood looking up for what felt like a lifetime, frozen to the spot and lost in the moment. As the last birds flew over my head, unaware of the incredible healing effect they had on me, the kettle, which was still struggling on the stove, began to whistle, signalling the task is complete.

Something about that moment had the power to lift me out of the feelings of crushing loneliness. I can't explain what it was, just that somehow I felt lighter, privileged to have been perhaps the only human at that moment to witness such a sight. Even thinking about it, I can remember that feeling.

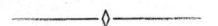

———◊———

That's what I'm looking for at Holkham today. I'm looking to recreate that emotion now in the hope that it will pull me away from the stress I've been under, the work that is piling up on my 'to do' list, the tasks I've been desperately avoiding. It all just feels a bit much at the moment. It's only January in 2024, and I'm struggling with this year already.

I get to the beach and it's freezing. A frosty breeze pushes its way through the tall pines, seeming to stop at my skin, making me instantly shiver as I press on to the sand sinking slightly in the loose surface. It's still light, a pink hue in the sky tells me the sun is starting to sink, and I stand for a while listening desperately to hear the sound that I've come here for. Twenty minutes pass and nothing. I'm shivering more dramatically now; the denim jacket was a poor choice but I left my 'Arsène Wenger' football manager's coat – you know, the long black puffer coats that seem to have risen to popularity – on the back of the sofa and this summer jacket was all I had in the boot of the car.

I decide to make the walk back to the car. Disappointed and still feeling rubbish, I turn and walk up the wooden stairs that lead from the sand back on to the boardwalk. As my foot touches the final step, a sound catches my ear and I turn. One lone pink-footed goose flies past. If there's one, there's likely to be more so I look in the direction the goose came from and, sure enough, more emerge from over the top of the pines. The sound gets louder and louder as more and more geese stream in over the trees. In front of me is a scene of awe and wonder.

The still sea and the pink sky act as a frame for the painting that is being drawn before my eyes as more geese are added to the picture, travelling quickly over the large expanse of wet sand. I feel lighter. I feel the anxiety fade, as though expelled from my body with each breath. A smile threatens to lift the corners of my mouth, and I realise how I must look to any dog walker passing by, freezing in a denim jacket on a Norfolk beach in winter, smiling at the sky. As the last geese fly out of sight, catching up with the group like passengers running for the last train at King's Cross, I trudge back through the pines towards the car feeling like I am ready to go home and take on the to-do list that awaits me. Instead of walking on the boardwalk this time, I deviate through on to the sand where the pines stand proudly and weave my way in and out of them. The sand beneath me looks like broken up chocolate chip cookies, pieces of wet black pine bark mixed in. I spot a razor clam shell sticking out of the cookie mixture, next to a pinecone. The long, white shape, synonymous with the beach, seems out of place in the trees. How did it get here? Did the wind carry it on a journey from the sea? Did an animal move it here after eating the creature within? Did a young child drop it on the way back to the car after spending a day splashing in and out of the waves? However it got here, it feels a little like our presence in nature. Somehow not quite right, but at the same time exactly where it needs to be. Two worlds meeting, the sea and the forest, two worlds that seem totally different and unsuited on first glance, but like Holkham, where pines blend with the beach, if you get it right, the perfect match.

At the car park, I sit at a circular picnic table for a while, not quite ready to go home yet. A pied wagtail lands on the table and sifts through some crumbs left over from someone's lunch. It hops around to face me and starts as it notices the giant sitting at the table. Sensing that I'm not a threat, it turns its back on me and continues to hoover up the carrot cake. Looking out across the field in front of me, I see a flurry of lapwings take to the sky in unison, magical colours shimmering as they swirl in a tornado of feathers. A breathy whistling sound is coming from a group of birds that look like brown ducks. Wigeon. For a long time, I thought *Wigeon* was just a misspelling of pigeon. These migratory ducks, which join us for the winter, fill the view in front of me and will be here to greet me every time I come back over the next few months. 'Wigeon city', my youngest calls it. Two greylag geese fly across the scene, angry honks sounding somehow less charming than their pink-footed cousins. They sound like they're complaining about something, perhaps the cold air that signals me to go home.

On the drive home, I pass a field full of another type of goose, a mainly black bird, smaller than a Canada goose, with a white 'dog collar' around its neck, making me think of a field of feathered vicars. A Brent goose. Another Arctic visitor to our shores during the winter months. The smallest of our geese and probably a species you may think is only accessible if you happen to live in a rural, east coast spot. However, I can assure you this is not the case.

## THE LIFE-AFFIRMING MAGIC OF BIRDS

The first time I saw this bird was in a much more urban location.

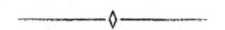

———◊———

February 2023 and I'm in Portsmouth. It's one of the most densely populated places in the UK, second only to London according to a 2021 census. Pulling off the motorway and driving towards the city, I go past a nature reserve which seems to encompass a vast marshland that runs into the sea where dozens of boats are moored, bobbing gently in the water. I look to the right as we pass a large playing field, and I doubletake as I see a group of large birds, black colour dominating against the white belly, huddled together in the middle of the grass.

*What on earth are they?* I ask myself.

A quick check on a bird ID app tells me they're brent geese. I haven't seen them before, and to see such a huge group standing together in the middle of a sports field where, at the weekend, the birds are replaced with football matches and picnics seems curious. Why do these birds, (13 per cent of the global population head to the Solent area, of which Portsmouth is part, I discover), which make their journey from Siberia, Arctic Russia, bypassing rural parts of the country, bypassing other brent geese which stop off in less built-up areas to spend their winter, travel all the way to Portsmouth, a densely populated, built-up concrete jungle?

Well, Portsmouth is technically an island, with extensive harbours and grass beds. Combine that with the abundance of grasslands in the area, and it provides the perfect place to feast for a winter season. These birds will have been travelling to Portsmouth long before humans moved in on the area, showing once again the adaptability and persistence of nature. As humans have encroached on this area, brent geese have continued to make the journey every year, determined not to be moved from their second home. I'd love to sit and have a chat with a brent goose. I'd like to ask how the landscape has changed. I'd find out if they have any tales from their ancestors about the Portsmouth of days gone by, before the huge naval bases were constructed, and before Charles Dickens was born in the old town. What was it like to be a goose before the amusements and chippies sprang up, before the schools and housing estates were built, before the human invasion? I wish we could sit down and hear their stories, but, alas, all we can do is listen to the storytellers who dedicate their lives to sharing stories on their behalf.

Oh, the things we can learn from these magnificent storytellers.

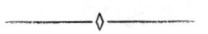

---------◊---------

Speaking of magnificent storytellers, sitting in front of me in a garden centre café on this May 2024 morning, a large cup of black filter coffee in front of him, is Nick Acheson. A writer and conservationist who literally wrote the book on geese, well, a book on geese. The book in question, *The Meaning of Geese*, is a beautiful retelling of a journey with the geese who come to Norfolk, as seen through the eyes of Nick and others who live and work alongside these long-distance visitors. The book's passion and love for the natural world is reflected in the man sitting in front of me today.

I don't remember how Nick and I first met, but I remember my first impression of him as one of astoundment. One, at the energy he gives off when talking about the natural world and, two, his unrivalled knowledge about what feels like everything that surrounds us. Nick tells me that, growing up in Norfolk, he was from a very outdoorsy family. He used to spend time trawling through brightly illustrated bird books, and a teacher at school turned him towards birds and showed him the magical world that he hadn't fully explored yet. With the help of his teacher, birds from his beloved books began to leap from the page, being brought to life in front of his eyes as he was introduced to a wonderful mixture of species that were available to him so close to home.

As we chat, Nick recounts stories of connecting with the pink-footed geese which he so fondly writes about. He shares my feeling that there is no better sound in autumn than a flock flying overhead in huge numbers and expresses disbelief that there are people who somehow manage to ignore it and not fling their heads back in absolute awe at the sound as they pass above us in the sky. But then again, until I moved to Norfolk, I didn't even like geese! Thinking of that time in my life doesn't fill me with regret or sadness or guilt at the fact I could have ever felt that way about such a fascinating group of birds. Instead, it reminds me of the importance of learning from those around us and listening to storytellers such as Nick, who are willing and ready to share their passion and knowledge with us when we are ready to hear it.

'I heard a willow warbler on my walk in today,' Nick tells me. I admit that I have never heard a willow warbler, or at least I don't know what they sound like. 'Right, let's go and hear one now.' Nick stands up, his excitement palpable. Obliging, I replace my coffee cup on the tray and follow him out of the garden centre and on to a small common that sits directly opposite and that I have somehow never noticed. Immediately the sounds of the birds fill my senses.

'Do you hear that one?' asks Nick, pointing towards a tall tree where a series of chirps dominate the chorus; this bird is definitely the lead singer. 'That's a song thrush. Collared dove: health and safety officers telling you to be careful.' Nick points towards the sound coming from a hedgerow and, sure enough, I can almost hear the bird forming the words 'be careful' as it calls from between the leaves. I watch and listen in total awe to this human who just radiates joy when he is surrounded by birds.

'Why do you love it all so much? Nature?' I am curious at what exactly it is that draws Nick into it.

'The world can just be so much bigger when you let nature in,' he replies, with pure magic in his voice, flinging his arms open as if welcoming the surroundings into his heart. 'Oh, there it is, the willow warbler. Listen.' He marches towards a different tree set against a small, concealed pond. A cascading trill falls slowly through the air as we listen carefully.

Nick continues to share with me a huge variety of treasures all within this one small patch of green space, surrounded by houses on all sides and a busy main road just a few hundred feet away. Nick puts his love for nature down to the fact he has fallen into the hands of people who know more than him and are willing to share their stories. Like him in this moment. And all I can do is listen and consider my gratitude for being in the presence of such a talented storyteller, one willing to share his tales with me.

And now, I hope, I'm bringing these stories to you for you to then pass on to someone else open to hearing them.

## THE LIFE-AFFIRMING MAGIC OF BIRDS

———◊———

I want to jump back in time now to 2023 to tell you about an unexpected, magical experience in nature that occurred on a very normal December day. The point is to remind you that these experiences can happen at any moment if you let them in.

The very first days of winter at Cley, my local nature reserve, just hits differently. I've often heard tales of the Taj Mahal being so unique in its colouring, that you can't actually photograph its true colour and you have to see it to understand its beauty for yourself. That's how Cley feels today, and no matter how hard I try and paint a picture for you now, it still won't be as breathtaking as it is as I stand here. Standing at the top of the East Bank, a long ridge that rises above the fields and channels that line either side, everything is still. And I mean really still. There isn't even the hint of a breeze moving the reeds today. The silence is almost eerie and yet there's something pure and magical about it. That magic of nature creeping in once again: you see a theme now? I hope you're almost convinced. The ground looks frosty, but it's not frost. It's not quite cold enough for that. It's a light dew that covers the bank on both sides, and the brightness of the day is bouncing off the tiny water drops, making them glisten like an avenue of ice.

The sky in front of me looks like a watercolour painting, as though the artist has dipped a paintbrush in a pastel pallet and moved from left to right leaving a wash of pinks and purples where the blue sky usually sits. I popped down for a quick walk after the school run, before getting started on the day's work. I never expect to see anything noteworthy, and yet every time I come here, I seem to spot something new. A bit like going into a clothes shop: there's always something new to see and try, fashions and trends changing with every season.

Walking along the bank, I stop to look at a swan which is moving slowly through a pool of water, surrounded by tall reeds. The pastel hue reflects perfectly in the water and makes the white plumage of the swan look brighter than ever before. As it glides gracefully through the water, the purple ripples following after it, the scene looks like a peaceful greeting card image.

I get to a channel which runs underneath the bank and stop at the wooden steps that lead down to the water. A few weeks ago, the kids and I stood just here with Nick Acheson as we waited in anticipation of an otter which had been seen that morning. Unfortunately, the otter was nowhere to be seen but Nick did tell me the signs to look for if ever I found myself here again. So, watching the still water, my excitement builds as I see ripples forming in the water. A coot shoots out of the reeds and proves to be the creator of the movement.

Not known for my patience, I turn to carry on walking but then an alarming sound comes from the water's edge. A high-pitched, squealing sound, like a pig in jeopardy. I've never heard this sound but based on Nick's spot-on bird call description, I recognise this as a water rail. Nick told me that if there are water rails (sculking birds of the reed beds with a bright red beak) chances are there's an otter nearby. I don't want to get my hopes up, but I decide to stay for another minute and see what happens.

## THE LIFE-AFFIRMING MAGIC OF BIRDS

A dark shape further down the channel is moving quickly towards me. Effortlessly swimming through the water and seeming to be dragging something behind it, the otter moves into view, pulling behind it the body of what looks like a goose. I stand statue still for fear of this moment being over before it begins. The otter seems to have reached its destination and begins to drag the goose into the reeds, and before long it gets to work on its breakfast. I move slowly down the steps in the hope of a better view. I've never seen an otter before and what if this is my only chance?

A woman in a bright yellow fleece with a border collie pulling her excitedly down the bank approaches and I gesture to her to be quiet and join me. She ties the collie's lead to the banister of the steps and moves quietly next to me.

'Wow,' she says quietly, 'I've never seen an otter.'

A man in a dark green raincoat with long Hunter wellies walks towards us from the other direction and we turn in unison, gesturing to him to be quiet. He obliges and says, 'Oh, wow,' slightly louder than I would have liked, but the otter doesn't seem to be bothered. It's too focused on its breakfast.

We stand for a while, three total strangers joined together by this moment unfurling in front of us. The air is still so still, I can hear the otter's teeth as it crunches through the bones of the carcass and plucks feathers from the skin. After around ten minutes, it drags the goose further into the reeds as though moving its bag of shopping into the kitchen to put it away for later. Then, it effortlessly slides underneath the surface of the channel.

'I suppose that's it then,' the yellow fleeced woman says, but then the otter reappears, moving up and down just in front of us, slipping in and out of the water, twirling in easy circles, like an eel. It moves with such ease and precision, it's clear this mammal is so perfectly adapted for the environment. After every tail flip and splash, the otter turns to look at us, as though it is watching the audience to gauge their reaction. I can't quite believe the scene that I am witnessing, and after another few minutes of the performance, I look at my phone and notice the time. I've got a meeting in half an hour. How would I explain being late? 'Sorry, I was watching an otter eating a goose and then putting on a show in the water in front of me.' Would they believe that or does it sound like a bit of a 'the dog ate my homework' excuse?

A series of events led to that moment. All of them coming together because of an exchange of knowledge. Nick initially brought me to this place, the location that otters had been spotted. He shared with me the signs and sounds to look out for. Signs and sounds that had once been shared with him and that he decided to pass on to me. The decision to come to this place to seek a little slice of tranquillity before starting work, and the hope that coursed through me as I stopped at that channel to try and spot my first otter. None of it would have been possible if we hadn't shared stories. And that man and woman most probably would have walked on by if I hadn't shared my experience.

Maybe you'll be able to go away from this chapter, look up the sound of a water rail squealing like a pig, and it will one day lead you to an otter. Perhaps next time you're at the park, instead of avoiding the geese, you'll see them in a new light and understand they're just doing what they can to protect their habitat. Possibly you'll hear the calls of a flock of pink-footed geese as you do your shopping in Formby town centre where they will pass over the Liverpool suburb on their journey, or you'll spot a playing field full of brent geese as you drive through the middle of one of the most densely populated places in the UK.

Whatever happens, take these stories with you and share them. Take your own stories and pass them around. You never know whose life you are enhancing by sharing your own knowledge and narrative. How much you can change things.

# 10
# ROOK

*'To thine own self be true.'*
– *Hamlet*, Act 1, Scene 2

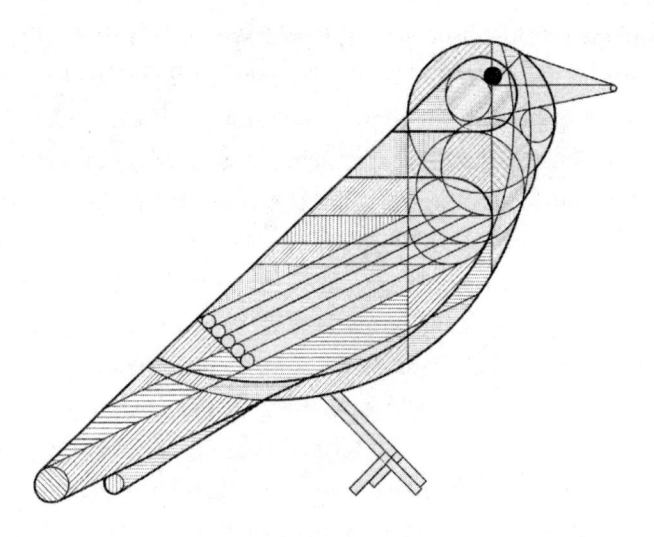

**There is beauty in the everyday**

If you stand in the playground of my kids' school, you are greeted by a row of towering Scots pines. Within these pines is a hub of chaos and activity – no trip to the school would be complete without hearing the squawks from the hundreds of rooks that call the trees their home. Well, for me, at least. These chatty birds often seem to be the root of much annoyance and inconvenience for other parents who, like me, spend an inordinate amount of time in that playground. These black birds often suffer mistaken identity. 'Those crows are loud today.' 'Oh my God, someone, please shoot those crows.' These are often phrases I hear as I stand beneath the trees, looking up and marvelling at this community of feathers living alongside the place where my children spend so much of their time.

Rooks are ridiculously intelligent birds. They belong to the corvid family, which includes crows, choughs, jays, magpies and the giant ravens, famed for guarding the Tower of London. You can tell rooks apart from their similar crow cousins, by looking for their naked patch of skin in front of their beaks. Rooks are extremely social birds, gathering in large groups, or rookeries, like the one at my kids' school. Their acrobatic aerial displays are quite a spectacle, and they fill the sky when coming in to roost, blocking out the sun with their sleek black feathers as they tumble and twist, greeting each other with their squawks and shrieks.

Rooks have a bit of a bad press in the countryside, but they play an important ecological role by controlling insect populations through their hungry snacking, spreading seeds and recycling nutrients with their scavenging habits. In other words, they're a really useful cog in a big environmental wheel. Just like every other species on our planet, they have evolved to fill an ecological niche, and without them we would observe major negative consequences. And we are lucky enough to have them here, at my sons' school, proving there's beauty in the everyday. If only we appreciate it.

---◊---

I'm standing in the school playground waiting for the kids to come out (for some reason my two are always the last) while other parents chat about the cold weather that's creeping in and the upcoming PTA event. The golden rays from the low sun paint the sky and I find myself staring up at the towering pines. It looks to me like the cover of a fairy-tale book; you know, the classic image of a magical forest where, inside, the lives of mystical creatures unfurl, unbeknown to the 'real' world. The breeze gently moves the needles of the pines, and the sound of the wind traversing through the branches provides a backing track to the late afternoon. I watch as the rooks begin to gather, a murmuration like a flock of starlings. Their movements seem so rehearsed as they meet in the sky, greeting each other after a day of scavenging and foraging in the fading light. It's a display of art as hundreds of birds move together in harmony, in total contrast to the harsh sounds coming out of their mouths. Corvids aren't known for their tuneful birdsongs. When research revealed that spending just six minutes surrounding yourself in birdsong can relieve anxiety, I don't think they were talking about the communal squawking of rooks.

They continue to circle above the playground, and yet somehow no one else seems to have noticed them, and I'm struggling to work out how not a single person is mesmerised by their performance. Their graceful efforts seem to defy gravity. 'God, that noise is awful,' one parent says who seems to have tuned in to their concert. I say nothing but, inside, my heart sinks a bit lower. As soon as they began, the birds start disappearing into the trees, perching on the ends of branches and selecting a perfect roosting spot.

A body slams into my leg and a bright yellow backpack is dumped heavily at my feet. 'No, don't go on the climbing frame, I want to leave,' but my frustrated voice falls on deaf ears as my youngest child runs off to the climbing frame with his friends.

The climbing frame is the bane of my existence; you'd think after six hours at school they would have had enough and be ready to leave the school gates. I look back at the trees and, lingering for a while, feel a deep, personal connection to the birds in front of me. For a split second it feels as though it's just me and them, bringing a sense of belonging to the wild world that many around me seem to have lost.

'Geeeeeese,' a familiar voice calls, growing louder as Jack, my eldest, hurtles towards me at full force.

'No, don't crash into me, please,' I say, automatically drawing my knee up to protect myself from his hulk-like strength.

'Look, *geese*,' he says again, pointing behind me.

I turn around and look at the eight greylag geese honking their way angrily past the school. The school run is, by default, boring. But these little experiences that I have allowed to creep into my everyday existence have a way of bringing a tiny, unexpected sprinkling of joy into the mundane. Noticing the riches that surround us has the power to turn the ordinary into the extraordinary.

The rooks in the trees seem to have got an undeservedly bad reputation. I personally think they're brilliant. Perhaps people view these birds with suspicion, associating them with ominous folklore or nuisance behaviour. Despite what are seen by many as negative associations, rooks are remarkably intelligent birds. Studies have shown that they possess problem-solving skills comparable to those of primates. Rooks are known to use tools to access food, such as dropping hard-shelled nuts on hard ground to crack them open, demonstrating both foresight and adaptability. They also exhibit complex social behaviours, living in large groups that cooperate and communicate effectively. You will have seen a rook, even if you haven't noticed it as such. You will definitely have heard them. You may have seen them and mistaken them for their crow cousins, as the parents do at my kids' school; their foraging behaviour often takes them to built-up areas, enlarging their communal rookeries and congregating in large numbers, and making their presence known to us humans with their chaotic chorus.

Ecologically, as I've said, rooks play a vital role in the well-being of our planet. As omnivores, they have a varied diet that includes insects, small mammals, seeds, fruits and carrion. By feeding on insects and small rodents, they help control pest populations. Their scavenging habits aid in the decomposition process, cleaning up dead animals and organic waste, which recycles nutrients back into the ecosystem. So, imagine a world without rooks for a moment. Without them removing the dead animals from our roadsides, they would quickly build up. Rooks are birds that play a crucial role in the ecosystem; like every species, they have their job in nature. Recognising their ecological contributions and shouting about their remarkable cognitive abilities can foster a greater appreciation for these often-overlooked members of the avian world. And I haven't mentioned their feathers yet.

A few weeks ago, I was walking back from my local shop in the rain, hood pulled over my head as the light shower slowly soaked me. In all the gentle rain, the lifeless form of a rook lay on the wet ground, wings outstretched as if in a final, silent flight. It looked like it had been hit by a car. I looked up and saw a rookery just above me, and it felt as though the group were looking down, mourning the death of their friend. Droplets of water clung to its still body, glistening like tiny jewels in the soft, diffused light. As the raindrops sat on the rook's feathers, the subtle iridescence of its plumage began to emerge, casting a spectrum of colours out into the world that danced with the light. Hues of deep purples, blues and greens shimmered, revealing the hidden beauty of the bird's glossy black feathers. Another unexpected display of nature's artistry highlighting the elegance often overlooked in the everyday. The rook, in life a symbol of mystery and intelligence, in death became a canvas. Each droplet refracted light, creating a mesmerising effect that transformed the scene from sombre to sublime, a reminder of the interconnectedness of life and death, and the extraordinary beauty that can be found in the most ordinary moments.

———◊———

Let's return to October 2021. We're in Wales and I've spotted my oystercatcher and I've begun to let nature weave its way back through my synapses, flooding me with that wild serotonin and starting me on my healing journey. The crisp mountain air whips around the parts of my face that are still exposed.

I'm standing in the car park of the National Trust's Ogwen Cottage. To my right there's a group of lads bending over their daysacks, checking their supplies; one has his head in the boot, rooting around for his other glove. It's a chilly morning and the air feels crisp. He will probably need that other glove once he gets some altitude. I close the door of my car, put my leg up on the wall and begin securing my boots.

'Alright?' He has found his glove and is now passing my car to begin his adventure.

'Hello,' I reply awkwardly. I've been so lonely for so long. A single parent, finishing a degree from behind my kitchen table as a global pandemic raged, and while two young children dance around the living room singing their own renditions of songs from *The Greatest Showman* and *Hamilton*, I've been so lonely. And yet here I am alone, experiencing a momentary connection with a total stranger. Two people connected for a brief second by a situation. Nature. I sometimes think we take these interactions for granted as you never know who is going to wander in and out of your life. Sometimes people turn up and stay. Sometimes, people flit in and out, perhaps to pay you a kind compliment that brightens your day, maybe to teach you a lesson about patience; whatever the reason, every interaction has the potential to be powerful.

I stop at a large information board which details the route up to Cwm Idwal, a hidden lake nestled below a gathering of rocky peaks. I pause here briefly; this isn't my first time visiting but I haven't been here long as a local resident. It feels different somehow; it feels like I'm a part of it now, old friends meeting up.

Following the constructed stone path which winds its way up gradually, I stop to look at the unmistakable shape of Tryfan, which casts its shadow across the valley. Sir Edmund Hillary climbed that very mountain in preparation for his attempt at summiting Everest. I try to imagine what it would feel like to stand on top of Everest, on top of the world. I can't. For now, what I can do is experience the gruelling hikes and scrambles of Snowdonia, the lactic acid building in my calf muscles, crying as I lose my way on an unknown ascent, smiling as I stand at the top.

When I arrive at the lake, the fog has descended, obscuring vision and creating an eery quiet broken only by the voices of a group just ahead of me on the path with a panting border collie straining to enter the water and splash in the shallows. For a while I just stand, looking out to where I know the lake is sitting under the thick blanket of damp cloud, breathing in the cold air and thinking of absolutely nothing. My mind is still, the pain of the last few years silenced.

As I perch on a solitary rock by the mist-shrouded shores of Llyn Idwal, letting the tranquil, obscured beauty of the landscape envelope me, the cloud moves, like someone rocking back and forth on their heels. The water, nestled amid the rugged peaks of the surrounding mountains, seems to shimmer ethereally in the soft light filtering through the dense fog. A scene of isolation, the peaceful kind, a sanctuary of solitude in among the chaos of everyday life.

A flash of movement catches my eye. A pied wagtail flits about in the mist. Its distinctive black and white plumage stands out against the grey backdrop, a beacon of life in the desolate landscape. I watch quietly as the wagtail dances gracefully in and out of the fog, its tiny and delicate form weaving through the damp air with ease. It seems completely at home in this remote wilderness, its presence a testament to the resilience of nature in the face of adversity. It strikes me that I've only ever seen these birds in urban settings. Instead of the mountainous backdrop, I've sat outside Starbucks and watched them move like clockwork toys around the outside tables. I've walked alongside one as I moved in and out of shops in a busy retail park.

As I observe the pied wagtail's solitary dance, I can't help but feel a sense of kinship with the tiny bird. Like me, it seems to find solace in the quiet beauty of this secluded corner of the world, seeking refuge from the noise and chaos of the outside world. It could be scuttling round one of the nearby towns. Llanberis, with its constant flow of foot traffic as tired hikers, coming down off the mountains, head to Pete's Eats for a bucket of coffee and a gigantic full English. I realise the huge impact that nature can have on our mental health, offering a sanctuary of peace and tranquillity in a world filled with uncertainty. The remoteness of this place, coupled with the presence of the pied wagtail, reminds me of the choice we have to take time for ourselves, to seek out moments of stillness and solitude in all the chaos. The bird has the choice to take flight and seek out 'greener pastures' and so do I.

As the fog starts to lift and the rays of sunlight begin to pierce through the mist, the pied wagtail bounces into the distance, leaving an empty rock where it once stood. I make my way back to the real world, taking with me a newfound appreciation for the healing power of nature and a lesson about the choices I have to make in order to take the necessary steps to remove myself from situations that don't fill me with joy anymore. Okay, this isn't black and white, but it's a rule I try and use in my life now. If it doesn't fill me with joy, then I don't need it. Amazing the epiphanies you can have when in the company of a bird that weighs the same as a couple of grapes.

Pied wagtails are charming little birds with black and white plumage. They're common across Europe, Asia and parts of Africa, and you will have encountered them in busy car parks, on rural nature reserves, moving like wind-up toys in the pursuit of dinner. The 'wagtail' part of their name comes from the long tail which it wags up and down to communicate with other members of the species. Like a lot of birds, they thrive in a range of environments and have adapted to urban life, making them a lovely feature in most cities. In the winter, pied wagtails can be found in big flocks, roosting together. In fact, the largest roost ever recorded was in a Kentish reed bed, where around five thousand individuals were counted. Like the rooks in my kids' school's trees, they're always there; we share our urban world with them. But how many people realise that? How many stop to look?

There was a pied wagtail scurrying around my feet on the day I went to visit the Cromer peregrines. I stood and watched while others marvelled at the birds of prey above us. Every day I look up at the sky as other school mums chat among themselves, ignoring the swirling black cloud of rooks circling above. These incredible moments occur around us every single moment of every day, but somehow we don't see them. I didn't see them either once, but when I did, the world around me suddenly became a much more vibrant, wonderful and awe-inspiring place.

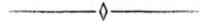

———◊———

It's January 2024. Stepping on to Holkham Beach once again, I am immediately struck by the vastness of the landscape that is stretching out before me. The sky seems to sprawl endlessly above, merging seamlessly with the horizon, while the sand below spreads out in all directions, a vast expanse of tiny grains rippling in the breeze. Trees twist individually, lining the distant dunes, their gnarled branches reaching towards the blue of the sky. Each tree tells a story of triumph, much like humans with our own personality and scars, shaped by our environment and experience. I can almost imagine the struggles they've endured, the battles against wind and weather that have left their mark upon their twisted forms. The sand flies across the beach like ghosts, swirling and dancing in the air before carrying towards the waves. It whispers past my ears, raw against my skin, causing my eyes to squint against the abrasive grains. Gritty eyes and crunchy teeth are the price I pay for the privilege of experiencing this untamed beauty. In the distance, ghostly snakes of wind slither towards the sea, churning through the sand, their ephemeral forms evaporating as they hit the water. Amid the swirling sand, sanderlings dart and weave, their tiny forms a blur against the whisps of sand kicked up by the wind. They seem to dance against the elements, fighting against the gusts that threaten to blow them off course. Every moment is a battle, a struggle for survival against the unforgiving forces of nature.

    I amuse myself with the horse prints etched into the sand, each a testament to the passage of time. I follow them along the beach, my footsteps echoing in the path they left behind them. I am a solitary figure in this vast landscape. It's a simple pleasure, tracing the path of another creature through this wild and raw wilderness. I wonder how many other footprints have been formed and washed away over the years. As I walk, I can't help but feel a sense of awe at the raw beauty of this place. The sound of the waves crashing against the shore is like a symphony, a soothing melody that washes over me, filling me with a sense of peace and tranquillity. The salty sea air invigorates my senses, filling my lungs with its briny scent. In this moment, I feel connected to something greater than myself, a part of the eternal dance of nature. And as I continue my walk along the beach, I carry with me a sense of gratitude for the simple pleasures of life – the feel of sand between my toes, the sound of the waves crashing against the shore, the beauty of nature in all its untamed glory. Revelling in moments like this that turn an ordinary day into a fairy tale.

My moment of clarity at Holkham couldn't last forever and I'm back in the school playground once again, searching for something to keep my mind busy. I blow out a sigh that's probably a bit too loud as I wait, slightly resenting the monotony of the school run. It often feels as though my whole life revolves around it, never quite having enough time during the day to get things done before I have to get in the car and be there to collect my children on time. *Is that a universal feeling among parents?* I wonder, as I lean against the wall where the empty house martin nest sits above me, waiting for warmer days when its residents will be back.

I prepare myself for the inevitable conversation that I'm about to have once my children emerge: 'No! Not the climbing frame, I want to get home.' 'Come on please you've been in school all day, haven't you had enough?' 'Right, I'm going, you can stay here if you want.'

The sky is cast in an inky shroud as I stand in the school playground, the air heavy with the promise of impending darkness. Lining the playground, the tall Scots pines loom, their branches stretching towards the heavens like outstretched arms. It's here, in the whispering pines, that the rooks roost, their caws and calls a familiar soundtrack to the school pick-up. A few other parents stand nearby, wrapped in coats against the chill of the evening. We exchange polite smiles and small talk: 'What you doing this weekend?' 'Swimming lessons tonight?' It's a routine we've grown accustomed to, these moments of waiting, forced together as our children pursue their extracurricular activities.

As we stand there, the conversation ebbs and flows, touching on everything from the weather to the latest school gossip. But then, Elaine, a grandmother with a sharp eye and a quick wit, breaks the monotony with a simple question that takes up all by surprise: 'Why is there a pheasant up that tree?'

Her words hang in the air, a curious puzzle that none of us can immediately unravel. We turn as one in the direction she's gesturing to, our eyes drawn to the silhouette of a lone tree against the darkening sky. And there, perched among the branches, is indeed a pheasant, its colourful plumage a stark contrast to the muted tones of the pine needles. For a moment, we're all silent, our minds racing to find an explanation for this unexpected sight. Then, all eyes turn to me, the 'bird nerd', 'bird woman'. I shrug, dumbfounded. I may like birds, but that doesn't mean I know why that pheasant is hanging out with my beloved rooks.

None of us can recall ever seeing a pheasant in a tree before, let alone one at such a height. It's a mystery that defies explanation, a small moment of wonder in an otherwise ordinary evening. But rather than succumb to confusion or frustration, we find ourselves united in curiosity, bound together by a shared sense of intrigue. It's a rare moment of connection, a reminder of the bonds that tie us together and to the nature that otherwise goes unnoticed in this playground.

We watch as the pheasant shifts its weight, its movements hesitant and uncertain. It's as if even the bird itself is unsure as to how it comes to be perched in this lofty position. And yet, there's a certain grace to its presence, a quiet dignity that commands our respect. As the minutes tick by, the sky darkens further and the pheasant shrieks its strangled chicken clucking sound. Still, we stand there, transfixed by the sight of this unexpected visitor in our midst. Noise grows as the kids erupt from school, their laughter and chatter breaking the spell of our shared reverie.

'No. Not the climbing frame. It's getting dark. I want to get home,' I cry at George as he deposits his bright yellow backpack at my feet and disappears up the slide with his best friend, Reed. Why do kids always walk up slides? I roll my eyes and look at Elaine, Reed's grandma, who, with a two-year old who keeps kicking off her golden cowgirl boots and writhing in the pram, I know feels the same about the climbing frame. My knees buckle as Jack crashes into me from behind. 'Suuuuuu,' he calls out, the Christiano Ronaldo goal celebration that seems to have become the song of eight-year-olds up and down the country.

'Right, I'm going. Stay here if you want, George,' I shout as I head towards the gate in a slow-moving herd with the other parents who are clamouring to leave. George launches himself down the blue plastic slide and collides with his friend, Wesley, who is lying on the ground beneath the slide waiting to be squashed by other users. Kids are weird.

With a final glance towards the tree, we adults all exchange knowing smiles, silently acknowledging the magic of this fleeting encounter. And as we make our way home, the memory of the pheasant in the tree lingers in the air, a gentle reminder of the unexpected joys that await us when we least expect them. The beauty that exists in the everyday.

# 11
# PARAKEET

*'It is not in the stars to hold our destiny but in ourselves.'*
*— Julius Caesar*, Act 1, Scene 2

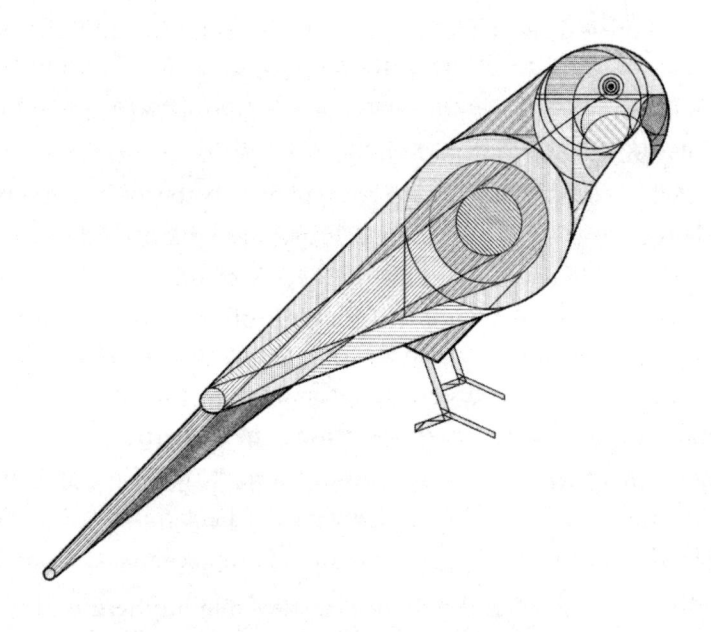

**Things change, that's guaranteed – it's up to you whether you choose to change with them**

October 2023. A green blur streaks in front of my eyes and I bend backwards, *Matrix*-style, maybe not quite, to avoid colliding with the shape. Half out of my car, I hold on to the open door as I watch it fly expertly across the car park and into the trees that line the perimeter. A sense of realisation dawns upon me and grinning like a fool, I say out loud to myself, 'Parakeet!'

I've been wanting to see a parakeet for ages. The number of times I've been around London and never seen them, or perhaps just never looked hard enough, and yet now, on my first proper, official 'nature outing' to the city, I am welcomed by a banner of colour. I'm at Walthamstow Wetlands, a London Wildlife Trust nature reserve in the borough of Waltham Forest, around seven miles from central London. This is my first real experience of a proper urban nature reserve. Well, my first purposeful trip to see birds in the middle of a city. I'm here to meet up with a group of people for an event I am leading for the birding app, Birda, one of several apps available out there that allow you to record your bird sightings an ID the things you are unsure of. On Birda the sightings are logged, then get translated into data that can help conservation scientists get a better picture of how bird populations are doing. I'd never used an app for birding before, but Birda drew me in because it's fun. It's bright and colourful, and there are always competitions and challenges to get you motivated to log what you find.

Over the last few years, I've had conversations with multiple individuals who don't seem to embrace the use of technology when it comes to nature. This is what I have to say to that: children, my own included, are spending more time than ever before behind screens, so it's a necessary evil. In fact, I reckon we are all spending perhaps a bit too much time on screens, if I'm honest. I get notifications every week to tell me how many hours I've spent on my phone and every week it shocks me. Whether I'm dead scrolling at night, or using my phone for work, my screen is very much a part of my everyday life. A 2019 survey reported that children under fourteen were spending about twenty-three hours a week using smart devices like phones, tablets and games consoles. It's easy to frisbee a tablet at the kids when they wake up with the sun, and it's a simple solution to let them play Fifa to their heart's content when I'm trying desperately to get work done in the evenings. Yes, I agree, I hate to see my kids sitting in front of screens and I do my best to direct them to educational content instead of watching ten hours of Mr Beast and his mates surviving on a raft in the middle of the ocean (a real video I suffered through with my eight-year old). But how is this for an idea instead of jumping to criticise all technology, should we not instead embrace the potential of it?

We are in a position where, for the first time in history, we can tap into a world of knowledge at the touch of a screen. My newfound curiosity for the natural world has only peaked because of the technology available to me. I know that if I walk past a plant and wonder what it is, I can just snap a quick picture, open up a plant ID app, and the information is there in front of me over and over again. We don't have to wonder what something is anymore, forgetting about it before we get home to look in a book. We can now enhance our knowledge on the go. Fast, take-away learning, yes, but learning nonetheless.

Every time my kids and I are outside, we take photos of flowers, fungi, insects, birds, mammal tracks, and we can instantly discover the identity of the species, information that we will retain and use again and again, in theory at least. In reality, my ability to remember plant species is beyond poor. The mystery of an unseen bird shouting at me from the hedgerows can be solved using an app. For me, it doesn't take away from the experience; in fact it makes the experience possible. I know full well, with the way my brain works, that I need the information like . . . now. If I have to remember what a leaf looks like and look it up at home, I will have forgotten the leaf exists by the time I even make it back to the car. But with the phone in my hand, I can be learning constantly. Yes, we need time without our devices. I actually love nothing more than being out of signal range for an afternoon on the local beach where I can spend a few hours fully immersed in the environment or with the people I am with. But, that said, technology is a tool we must use to empower ourselves as we move forward with the fight for the natural world. If a kid is using a phone to identify the call of a bird in the middle of the woods, surely that's better for the future of the species around us than a kid ignoring their surroundings.

A point on social media, too: it has its bad points. Boy, does it have its bad points. But using social media platforms has allowed me to connect with people from all over the world whom I may not otherwise have had the chance to speak to. It's given me the chance to learn from the most brilliant and experienced naturalists, creating opportunities that I never thought were accessible to me.

We are at a crucial crossroads in our environmental history. We are faced with two options. Option A, we carry on this path of destruction, destroying landscapes and taking countless species down with us. Or Option B, we can start using whatever methods we have available to deconstruct barriers brick by brick, showcasing the natural world to as many people as possible and highlighting the beauty that is all around us if we only look for it. Britain has lost 73 million birds in the last fifty years, a number that is set to rise. The *State of Nature Report*, compiled by sixty nature organisations, concluded that one in six of UK species are at risk of extinction, largely due to anthropogenic effects. The UK is one of the most nature depleted countries in the world and we have lost over half of our native biodiversity. Millions of birds are missing from the skies. This is a fact that we have to face, and we must use our knowledge, passion and power – however we get it, with whatever tools at our disposal – to help those around us begin to notice nature, whether that's venturing to a nature reserve to encounter rare migrants or opening the back door and stepping into a garden.

The more people engage with nature in whatever means available to them, the more chances we have to share and disseminate knowledge. Next time you're outside, be it in a city or in the middle of nowhere, whip out your phone and snap a dodgy picture of a bird or a weird looking leaf. Find out what it is. Share it with a friend. Let's make noticing nature fun and continue to build a community of individuals who are furiously determined to create a world where we live in harmony with wildlife. Remember, we don't own this planet; we are as much a part of nature as the birds on your feeders, the berries ripening in the hedgerows. It begins with looking outside and flying through the gateway to nature. All it takes is a change of mindset. The world is moving. It's up to you whether or not you move with it.

———◊———

I'm at Walthamstow Wetlands, standing by a large body of water, waiting for the Birda group to arrive. A huge row of towering flats line the view, reminding me how close I am to the human world. The group is made up of naturalists, birders and people who, like me, are new on this journey to reconnecting with nature, and to be honest, I cannot wait to spend the day in the company of people who just get it. Who won't judge me if I stand and marvel at one of the many species of birds I'm about to see. Who won't laugh at my astonishment at the amount of species we spot so close to the capital city, and who will join me as I lie on the ground to snap a photo of a fly. (Wait, doesn't everyone do that?)

As I wait, I watch a cormorant land on the island opposite me, joining several others standing like tiny dragons with their wings outstretched. For a bird that spends its life diving effortlessly in and out of the water to catch its dinner, cormorants skipped a vital evolutionary step and don't possess the ability to create the waterproofing substance used by other seabirds to keep them dry during their semi-aquatic lives. Though if they did have this oil in their feathers, they wouldn't be able to swim with such ease through the water, like feathered fish. This is why you'll always spot cormorants hanging out like dragons with their wings outstretched while the wind dries their feathers.

A man with his hood pulled up over his head, and looking like he is a walking advert for Nike, moves towards me, a huge bully dog running freely off the lead. Being a dog lover, I put my hand out to the dog and say 'hello' as she barrels towards me to greet me. The man, pulls his hood down and I see a young face etched with nerves as he speaks to me.

'She's proper friendly, I promise, she wouldn't hurt anyone.' I think he is nervously protecting himself and his dog as he remembers the proposed legislation to put a muzzle on bull breeds over a certain size, and looking at this dog, she definitely falls into that category.

'It's fine, I love dogs. She's beautiful.' I kneel down to her level and let her place her head gently on my shoulder. He relaxes and we chat for a while.

'You looking at birds?' he asks, pointing at the binoculars around my neck.

'Yes!' I reply eagerly. 'It's my first time here and I've seen so much already.'

'Cool innit, I always see them dragons. *How to Train Your Dragon* vibes,' he points to the cormorants. 'Dunno what they are though.' I explain to him what they are and why they all have their wings outstretched.

'Cool, never knew that.' And whether he will pass that information on to anyone else or keep it to himself, I feel good to have had this chat and shared a little bit of something with a stranger. Maybe it won't change his world in the way nature changes mine every day, but perhaps on his daily dog walk through the site, he will look at those birds and remember a conversation with a stranger and a brief connection to something unknown, something exciting, something that's just there waiting.

Parakeets, also known as ring-necked parakeets or rose-ringed parakeets, are a colourful and charismatic, or annoying depending on whom you speak to, species of bird that have become a familiar sight in London and now throughout the United Kingdom. Native to parts of Asia, these birds were introduced to the UK through a combination of accidental releases and deliberate escapes, and they have since established thriving populations in various parts of the country. The story of how parakeets came to be in the UK is still up for debate, but there is no doubt that it's rooted in a combination of human activity and natural adaptation. While there are some arguments over the exact origins of the UK's parakeet populations, it is generally believed that the birds first arrived in the mid-twentieth century as a result of the exotic pet trade.

There are a few urban legends surrounding their origins, though, of course, in true legend style, none of them are supported by any actual evidence. Perhaps my favourite myth suggests that parakeets were introduced by musician Jimi Hendrix in the 1960s. According to this story, Hendrix released a pair of parakeets into the skies of London as a symbolic gesture of peace and love during one of his concerts. While it's true that Hendrix did own a pair of parakeets during his time in London, I haven't found any truth in that story.

Another commonly heard myth is that parakeets were brought to the UK by film crews during the filming of John Houston's *The African Queen*, a film made in the 1950s. The story goes that parakeets were used in the film and were subsequently released into the wild after filming was completed. Still prefer the Hendrix theory.

In reality, the true origins of parakeets in the UK are less interesting. Parakeets are escape artists and can easily slip out of cages if given the opportunity. I mean, wouldn't you? Once released into the wild, they are capable of thriving in a variety of habitats and climates, which has allowed them to establish populations in many parts of the UK. Adaptable little green friends, well, to me at least. The presence of parakeets here has sparked some controversy, particularly among conservationists concerned about their potential impact on native bird species, yet many people have come to appreciate these colourful birds as a unique and welcome addition to the country's wildlife.

The story of parakeets in the UK is another testament to the resilience and adaptability of nature. Despite their origins thousands of miles away, these charismatic birds have found a home here, where they continue to delight with their colourful plumage and lively antics.

———◊———

I'm in London again. It's April 2024 and I'm here to see Dr Sean McCormack again. Well, after taking me to see peregrines at Ealing Hospital, I went back to soak up more of his knowledge and learn about some of the other interesting projects that are going on within the borough. One of which surprised me.

*Beavers in London.* Surely not? I'm still in half-disbelief that I'm on my way to explore the Ealing Beaver Project with Sean.

Even the name doesn't sound right to me.

Ealing, a bustling borough, full of roadworks, grey tower blocks, busy restaurants and lorries fighting their way through the streets to get to the outlying industrial estates. Beavers, an animal I associate with North America and can think of the number of cartoons I've sat and watched with the kids where an American beaver features. They're just not a species I've ever considered as being here in the UK. Beavers were actually once native to the UK and were hunted to extinction in the sixteenth century for their fur, meat and castoreum – yes, that is their scent gland fluid in case you were wondering.

In recent years, there have been efforts to reintroduce them into certain areas as part of conservation projects. Their presence can have significant ecological benefits, such as creating habitats for other wildlife, improving water quality and reducing flooding. Despite some controversy over their reintroduction, beavers are gradually making a comeback in the UK, showing the focus and the importance of restoring balance to ecosystems and preserving biodiversity.

I park my car at Greenford Station, squeezing into the last remaining space between another car and a wall. I realise this space has multiple uses when I get out and the smell of urine hits me, but I've found a parking space so I'm not going to complain. Sean told me to head for a retail park and to find an underpass, and to be quite honest, I really can't imagine what I'm about to experience. I still can't quite work out how beavers fit into this truly urban environment. I walk past a busy McDonalds, workmen and families enjoying a meal with coats pulled up around themselves against the chilly air.

Having experienced plenty of dodgy feeling underpasses, I prepare to carry myself quickly through a dark tunnel littered with rubbish and cigarette butts. As I approach said underpass, the anxiety lifts as I see solid metal gates beckoning me towards a bright and airy space. Inside are walls decorated with the most spectacular mural. A giant kingfisher welcomes me, a newt floats along the painting and, of course, illustrated beavers look back at me as I walk, seeming to point the way.

'There's another mural just round the corner if you like this one,' a man with a caramel Labradoodle says as he stops next to me while I marvel at the artwork.

# PARAKEET

The underpass tells me I'm heading to somewhere truly unique, and walking through the metal gate at the other end of the tunnel, I emerge into another world. The busy retail park that lies just behind me feels a million miles away. The sound of the road is muffled by the swaying trees whose leaves rustle gently. Blackbirds and blue tits sing from within their branches and a wren performs its machine gun-like trilling from somewhere on the grassy ground. The tarmac path seems to disappear into a thick jungle of evergreens, and I keep walking towards a signpost that I have spotted. It bears the words 'Ealing Beaver Project' in a unique graffiti-style artwork which seems to pay homage to the urban world sitting just a few steps away.

Sean waves and greets me and we walk together, him pointing out wildlife cameras hidden in the shrubbery and strapped to trees. We stop at a small pond surrounded by bullrushes with bad haircuts, like huskies when they shed their fur. A pair of runners come past us and smile a 'hello', which feels unusual for London. Perhaps it's the natural influence filling them with joy, so much so, they've broken the 'norm' of the city and greeted two strangers. A wren calls again from somewhere low down, seeming to have a sort of rap battle with a woodpigeon which calls out its familiar tune.

I spot one of the concealed wildlife cameras strapped to a tree and wonder how many times my feet have been unknowingly captured as I've walked so far. The unmistakable call of a peregrine sounds from above me. I wonder if it could be Dusty or Freddie, the peregrines from Ealing Hospital. Or could it be another individual passing through on the hunt?

## THE LIFE-AFFIRMING MAGIC OF BIRDS

Sean leads me back to a group of people who are here for one of the popular Beaver tours that he leads here, this one from an organisation called Trees for Cities, a charity that does exactly what it says on the tin and helps local communities to plant trees in urban areas. To date, they've planted over 1.7 million trees, both in the UK and internationally, and this group in front of me is part of that effort.

Each one of them is excited and passionate about creating greener spaces and giving people access to trees. Sounds good to me. They seem to buzz with anticipation to see the project and Sean leads us to a stream which winds its way under the path and out the other side. He points towards a pile of thin branches which look to have been deliberately placed across the stream of water, slowing the flow. This beaver dam is creating a pond where the beavers can hide in the deep water, if needed. I always assumed (not that I'd spent much time thinking about it) that beavers lived in the dams they create. But Sean tells us that the reason they create these dams is for these deep beaver ponds which allow the creatures to have a safe space to shelter from predators and to raise their young. They will then build a lodge within the pond which becomes their home, where they can sleep and keep warm. The dams they create contribute to a wider ecosystem by creating wetland areas that can help other species thrive.

Quickly changing into my wellies, I join the others and follow the stream off the main path and down a muddy grass track to a second dam, where we stop. Sean tells us about a trip to Bavaria where he went to visit a German beaver population and witnessed the full potential of their engineering capabilities when he saw a dam that was around a quarter of a mile long. As well as creating themselves a home, the dam acted as a multi-species housing development, with voles burrowing, snakes nesting and plants taking root within the structure. It's as though the beavers are the architects, creating new housing for those with whom they share the space.

As I study this small dam in front of me, I can see shoots where the willow is trying to push through and grow, a living world within the structure. The beavers have only been here in Ealing for four months and yet they've created four dams, meaning they're already helping to create an ever-expanding ecosystem.

Jon Staples is a ranger who works alongside Sean on the beaver project and at other green spaces in the borough. We hang at the back of the group, his well-behaved border collie staring up at me, begging to be stroked, which I willingly do. Jon tells me that he worked as a youth worker for the council when a ranger job came up and he jumped at the chance.

'Would you ever change the work you do now?' I ask, wondering if he would move away from this job now he's discovered it. He thinks about it for a second, looking at the beaver dam. 'I'd like to do a bigger and more challenging project,' he says after a while.

'Bigger than releasing beavers in London?!'

He laughs and tells me that there's so much that can be done; the beavers are just the beginning. He tells me that he learns from the beavers, applying techniques they use for managing water flow and water clarity to other sites he works at. It feels wonderful to spend a few minutes talking to this man who has truly found his place and knows exactly where he is meant to be. He spotted an opportunity and he went for it, and now spends his days learning from another species about managing the land he works on. Of course, learning from each other needn't be limited to just humans. Other species have survived in their habitats for a lot longer than we have, developing ways to use the landscape to suit their needs without causing a negative knock-on effect and, I hope you'll agree, we could do with taking a leaf out of their book.

I ask Sean about the reception people have given the beavers, as it must seem an odd thing to have them in such an urban area, to which he replies that people in urban environments have less access to nature, so give them more and they readily welcome it: 'People are excited by it.'

'Look,' Sean quietly shouts, beckoning the group to the edge of the path and pointing at the ground. He is standing by a bright yellow sign which announces, 'beavers crossing', set against a backdrop of a grey high-rise building. It shouldn't work, but somehow nothing has ever seemed more right.

I move to look and see a trail of large footprints framing the edge of the path and leading back towards the water. 'God, they're big.' I'm not sure I've ever considered how large a beaver's feet might be, but aligning my lime green wellie alongside one of the elongated footprints, it seems that this particular beaver was around a size six.

Sean and I bid farewell to the group at the end of the tour, everyone feeling wholesome and happy to have seen something so wonderful. I head back to my car ready to head to my next wildlife destination, Sean's flat.

Stopping off at a shop to grab some lunch, I spend five minutes sitting behind a very shiny Mercedes which is waiting for a particular parking spot, despite there being two other spaces available. As I wait, I look out of the car window and see a parakeet swinging off a bird feeder at the front of a red brick house. It still seems odd to see these tropical looking birds hanging off the front of a 1950s English house, but at least they bring a bit of colour to the moment as the Mercedes finally gets the desired parking space.

I pull up at Sean's building, and after buzzing the wrong flat and having to call him, I wait to be buzzed in. An odd noise comes from next to my feet and I look down to see a round, ginger cat; it sounds like it is auditioning (badly) for the cello part in an orchestra. The door opens and, seconds later, I find myself in Sean's apartment looking at the very thing I came here to see.

Okay, let's step back for a brief second and address the elephant in the room, or the parakeet in London in this instance. Obviously, parakeets aren't native to the UK. We've talked about the many theories about how they got here, but I couldn't write about them without touching on the negative comments when you mention a parakeet. And that's why I wanted to talk to Sean about this. Sean is a vet, a birder, a naturalist, a campaigner and, most importantly for me, balanced.

I ask Sean what he thinks about this non-native, escaped species which has so successfully colonised parts of the UK and seems to be spreading across the country. Sean tells me that the jury is out on the negative impact that parakeets have on our native bird species. They are cavity nesters, finding holes in trees and buildings to raise their broods, and they do displace birds from nesting sites. Smaller species like tits are losing out to the bigger, bulkier and more aggressive green birds, for sure. People see them dominating bird feeders and hoovering up all of the seeds, but Sean says, 'putting feeders out for the local birds isn't exactly natural, is it?' I've never thought about it like that, and that's what Sean does: makes you think about things that you may never have considered.

Sean's view on the matter is they do have an impact but they are here, so we deal with it. He tells me that they have been around for over half a century now and there seems to be no joined-up thinking as to what to do about it.

'A species gradually reaches critical mass and then sort of explodes,' he explains, 'and that's what's happened now as we see them spread out of London as far up as Bradford now.'

'But,' I add perhaps naively, 'it's not their fault, they just made the most of a situation.'

'No, that's true,' Sean backs me up, 'and there seems to be a changing narrative around non-native species and some people are referring to it as "new nature".'

We talk about the biodiversity crisis, and Sean explains that as he sees it, everything is in a free fall, one in six species of plant and animal in Britain threatened, but then you have species that are doing really well. There seems to be a shift in thinking, saying we should be celebrating the success stories, the species which seem to be thriving in our massively altered ecosystem. We've created a new nature and species are able to fit into ecosystems that they wouldn't have before. I wonder if that's challenging to accept, as a conservationist where the narratives all seem to be around preserving and restoring what once was.

I've never considered that the world is a very different place to the world of fifty, one hundred, one thousand years ago. Perhaps we can't recreate that exact world; perhaps we are moving towards a new world.

'I've found it difficult, yeah,' Sean replies with no hesitation. 'As a conservationist, naturalist, biologist, whatever, you're taught the traditional narrative that non-native species are bad. But we are working with an ecosystem that is entirely different to anything we have seen before. Species are naturally moving in and starting to take hold.'

'Yes, parakeets are a different story, they were released, but we've transported plants and animals all over the world and London itself has become a big melting pot of species.' He gestures out of the window at the view, a line of tall, diverse trees where two parakeets pick at the blossom. The scene looks like something out of a tropical painting.

'Half of these trees that you can see aren't native, but we live with them and even celebrate them.' He gestures to the large wooden nest box tucked on to his balcony. 'This causes split feelings. People ask why I'm providing a nesting space for pests.'

No one has ever stuck a camera inside a parakeet nest, and so Sean and wildlife wonder Kate McCrae have done just that. This nest box is here in the hope that we can observe a parakeet nest for the first time to help us understand the species a little bit more.

'Look at the male,' Sean points at one of the parakeets, 'he's got that ring going all the way around his neck, lilacs and pinks, whereas she hasn't got as much of a ring.' He hands me a pair of binoculars, but the bright ring is so vibrant, I can see it without.

Sean goes on to tell me about the peregrine box at Ealing Hospital, and how they've seen an increase in parakeets making up a portion of the peregrine's diet. I suppose their distinctive screeching and their bright colour make them an easy target for an apex predator like a peregrine.

'Hey, have you ever seen a kingfisher in London?' Sean asks me, changing the subject.

'No, I literally never see kingfishers. They're like unicorns, I think,' I reply.

'Come on then, I bet you I can show you a kingfisher.' Unconvinced, I follow Sean outside for yet another adventure.

The screech of the parakeets is loud by the river; green shapes stream back and forth over our heads and we follow them to where they seem to be landing. A dead tree trunk, around twenty feet tall and chopped off at the top, stands to the side of the muddy path. In the trunk I can see a series of perfectly rounded holes, like windows, placed sporadically up and down the trunk. As we watch, a parakeet sticks its head out of one of the holes and another lands at the entrance to the hole, in a kind of Uber Eats-style food delivery. The scene is repeated in a hole just above, and the more we look, the more of the vibrant birds seem to be nesting in the tree.

The scene reminds me of a block of flats, each flat containing a family who are going about their lives, shouting at their neighbours if they get too close. This block of flats, instead of being a grey stone building, though, reminds me of the Great Elf Tree from Ben and Holly (parents of young kids, you'll know exactly what I mean).

We move round to the river's edge where a huge collection of dead trees, branches and, sadly, litter, have collected, forming a mass that slows the flow of the water.

'It looks like your beavers have been here and built a dam,' I say, sadly observing the plastic containers, rope, crisp packets and general foamy sludge that have congregated in an ugly mass.

'There's a kingfisher,' Sean interrupts quietly, pointing at the bank opposite. And sure enough, just for a split second, I see a metallic blue ball sitting on a branch that is overhanging the flowing water.

'Told you,' Sean says smugly.

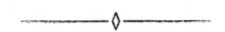

---◊---

I've always loved Tudor history, and as I step through the ornate gates of the 500-year-old Hampton Court Palace, and into the large courtyard, I'm transported back in time from May 2024 to 1537, when Jane Seymour gave birth to a future king here. I feel like all of the history lessons from school and countless episodes of *Horrible Histories* come to life in front of me. The opening number to *Six: The Musical*, the modern retelling of the six wives of Henry VIII, plays on a loop in my head. The grandeur of the architecture surrounds me, its imposing stone walls and towering turrets speaking of centuries of stories passed down through the bricks. I can't help but feel a sense of awe as I make my way towards the entrance, each step echoing with the weight of the past.

Hampton Court was gifted to Henry VIII in the 1520s by Thomas Wolsey, Archbishop of York, and Henry clearly saw in it the same beauty as I do, with its close proximity to the river and then large hunting grounds surrounding it, now known as Bushy Park. He got the Tudor *Grand Designs* in and extended it into an even larger palace, his favourite of all his residences, and brought all six of his wives here – not at the same time, of course. It was passed from royal to royal, and the back of the palace was remodelled by none other than Christopher Wren (of St Paul's Cathedral fame, who also redesigned around fifty-two churches in London after the Great Fire of 1666), when William and Mary commissioned Fountain Court, a baroque remodelling in 1689. I'm only thankful that Wren left the magnificent Tudor front to the palace when he tore down some of the original apartments to remodel; otherwise, we'd be looking at a very different palace.

Entering the palace is like stepping into a living museum. The opulent furnishings and intricate tapestries tell the story of a bygone era, where kings and queens ruled with absolute power and authority. It's a fascinating glimpse into a world long gone, and I find myself lost in the grandeur of it all as I stop at a portrait of Anne Boleyn, Henry's second wife. I wish the portrait could speak to me. I have so many questions about what life was actually like in the Tudor courts. Imagine having a first-hand account without our twenty-first-century interpretations.

I recall reading a debate on Instagram lately (my algorithm knows me well) about a letter which was penned by Henry's fifth wife, Katherine Howard, to her presumed lover, Thomas Culpepper, which formed some of the evidence in her execution trial. Some people in the comments section were hell-bent on this being a love letter; some regarded it as more of a business transaction. Either way, it's a bit like in GCSE English Literature when you have to analyse why Dickens used the colour blue to describe the sky – we will never really know, and perhaps the sky was just blue that day? It's also a bit like what Sean McCormack said about nature. Things have changed so much in the last 500 years, whether we are talking about life in a Tudor court or an ecosystem. Things are dramatically different and we can't simply look at things through our modern lens without consideration of that fact.

After a quick tour of the palace – we always tour historic houses at record breaking speeds, the kids asking approximately thirty thousand questions each and my knowledge and ability to answer the questions slowly running out as we head towards the more modern parts of the building – George, my youngest, stops in the Hanoverian room (the period between 1714 and 1837, when there were a lot of King Georges who originally came from, you guessed it, Hanover). He lingers by a portrait of George III, his favourite king (well, we all have one, right?), the longest reigning British king ever and famed for being 'mad'. His real reason for this favouritism lies in the musical *Hamilton*, in which George III makes an appearance.

A friendly room guide suggests we have a 'George' photoshoot and encourages my son to pose in the same way as the many portraits of the many Georges, which, naturally, he does with enthusiasm. We eventually step outside into the palace gardens, and I'm truly taken aback. The air is alive with the sound of birdsong, a symphony of chirps and trills that fills the breeze with music. We head towards the long 'canal' which was commissioned by Charles II for his new wife, Catherine. They honeymooned at the palace and boats in the shape of swans sailed up and down in celebration. Today, there are no swan shaped boats, but a pair of actual swans glide gracefully up and down, arguably better.

A familiar screeching noise sounds overhead, and we follow the sound towards an avenue of trees where a riot of colour catches my eye. There, in the verdant foliage, I catch a glimpse of the parakeets. Their vibrant plumage stands out against the lush greenery, a splash of emerald and pink in a sea of leaves. I can hardly believe my eyes as I watch them flit about, their wings beating in a blur of motion as they dart from branch to branch. I suppose I just wasn't expecting to see these tropical birds in the grounds of Hampton Court. I wonder what Henry would have made of these loud birds. Actually, knowing Henry VIII, he probably would have tried to hunt them and display them in the palace.

I've seen parakeets loads of times now, dangling off feeders and snacking on blossom, but I've never seen them up close before. Here, they hang confidently on the low-hanging branches, unfazed by people walking past and taking photos. They're much larger than I expected, their size and majesty taking me by surprise. We watch them, mesmerized by their beauty and grace as they go about their business, seemingly unperturbed by our presence.

As I watch, one of the parakeets sits on a nearby branch, its bright eyes fixed on me with a curious gaze. It seems to be studying me with as much interest as I have in it, before it lets out a cheerful *SCREECH* and glides on to the wind. Eventually, I tear myself away from the parakeets and continue my exploration of the palace gardens. But the memory of that encounter stays with me, a reminder of the unexpected joys that await us when we take the time to appreciate the beauty of the world around us.

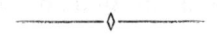

---

St James's Park is quite possibly one of my favourite places in the world. I know I haven't seen and experienced the whole world yet, but in terms of places I've been so far, it is one place

## PARAKEET

I always come back to. The park is located in the heart of London, sitting just in front of Buckingham Palace. Like a lot of the city, it has a rich and interesting history dating back as far as William the Conqueror, who was one of a series of owners of the land. A marshy area that was used for hunting and grazing pigs by Henry VIII (there he is again), the park came into some semblance of what we know today when Henry built the hunting lodge that would eventually morph into the palace that still stands today. A hospital for women with leprosy, the Leper Hospital of St James the Less, was always situated on the site and gave the park its name.

The land was drained and transformed into a royal park by King James I in the early seventeenth century. He kept exotic animals like camels, crocodiles and an elephant, and created pools that became the ponds that are still there today.

Over the centuries, it has served as a backdrop for numerous royal events and ceremonies, including royal processions and celebrations. Don't forget, during all this time, Buckingham Palace wasn't the palace we know today. It was bought in 1761 by George III (there he is again), and throughout the early nineteenth century, St James's Park underwent a series of renovations under the direction of landscape architect John Nash, who was responsible for the extension of Buckingham Palace and who transformed it into the picturesque landscape we know today. The iconic lake at the centre of the park was created during this time, providing a tranquil oasis among the hustle and bustle of the city.

Throughout its history, St James's Park has been a destination for Londoners and tourists alike, offering an incredibly biodiverse and peaceful retreat from the chaos of urban life. Today, it is home to an array of flora and fauna, including over forty species of waterbird, some of them 'collection' birds, but also species like coots and a whole range of weird and wonderful ducks which call the ponds their home.

Perhaps the most notable species for visitors to the park are the pelicans. Yes, pelicans. I knew nothing about them the first time I visited, and crossing over the road from Horse Guards Parade to join a gathered crowd to see what was going on, I did a double take when I saw three huge, pink pelicans standing in front of me. One greeted me by opening its huge bill and spitting out a pile of brown leaves by my feet.

The pelicans have been there since 1664 when they were presented to Charles II. Obviously not the exact same pelicans, but there have been pelicans in the park since the Merry Monarch's days. The one thing that always amazes me in St James's is, no matter who you are, whether you're into nature or haven't converted to birdwatching yet, the birds are so abundant in this relatively small area, you have no choice but to take notice. I've sat on a bench surrounded by pigeons like that pigeon woman scene from *Home Alone*, and watched tourists marvel over the species, like the greylag geese, which they might never have seen before.

I've seen gilet warriors – young blokes in tailored suit trousers, white shirt sleeves perfectly rolled up who have clearly stepped straight out of the Financial District – deep in conversation with colleagues, break their conversation to say, 'Look at that weird duck.' No matter who you are, St James's is a place that draws you close to nature, and in such close proximity to the busiest parts of the city, it still surprises me to have such a haven in a seemingly heartless world. Yes,

## PARAKEET

I know a lot of the birds are non-native, collection birds. And yes, I know that actual birders don't 'count' the birds in St James's Park.

I've trawled through birdy forum discussions full of people encouraging others to ignore the wildfowl of central London, and whatever you do, don't include them on your tick lists. But, at the end of the day, if there is a space where birds are living freely and the general public, possibly some of them for the first time in their lives, can connect in some way to them, does it really matter?

As I stroll through St James's Park with my mum and the kids, the hustle and bustle of the city fades away, replaced by the soothing sounds of nature. We are on the way to the theatre to take the boys to their first ever West End musical, an emotional day for me, who started off life as a theatre kid. We could have taken the tube; it would have been quicker. But given the chance, we will always choose to walk through this park, taking a slow meander past the ponds to visit the geese and say 'hello' to the squirrels.

The air is alive with the chatter of birds and tourists, their melodic songs filling the air with music – the birds, not the tourists. As we wind our way along, a group of people dressed as dragons, paper costumes rustling as they walk, stroll past us, chanting a poem, some of them twirling as they go. No one bats an eyelid as they pass. *London*.

We stop at the low black railing which separates us from the large ponds and watch as a flock of pigeons accost a woman who is trying to eat a sausage roll. Her family look on, laughing, and taking photos instead of coming to her aid. I hear that squawk and look up to see three parakeets hanging upside down on the branches above us, their colourful plumage glowing against the backdrop of the park. I can't help but smile at the sight, feeling a sense of joy at meeting these birds which now feel like old friends. Without hesitation, and remembering something a friend told me last time we were here, I dig around in my bag and find an apple which has seen better days. I bite into it – yep, it definitely has seen better days – and give it to George, my youngest, and the one who is the most 'nature friendly' out of the two.

He holds it out towards the parakeets. They regard him with cautious interest, their beady eyes fixed on the offering in his hand. And then, as if sensing that we mean them no harm, they begin to approach, their movements hesitant at first, then growing bolder with each flap of the wing as they move on to lower branches. Before long, a parakeet lands on George's arm and begins to have a go at the apple. I study the parakeets up close, their dazzling plumage a glorious display of nature's beauty. A couple of others hover nearby, their wings outstretched as we move pieces of apple to the fence, where they pounce.

For a moment, watching these birds here, I forget that I'm in the middle of a capital city.

'Why is that goose up a tree?' Reluctantly I tear myself away from the feeding station and look at where my mum is pointing. An Egyptian goose (which is actually not a goose, or a duck as it turns out – I don't think it really knows what it is, it's just an Egyptian goose) is staring down at us from a thick branch above our heads.

'Hmm, I've never seen a goose up a tree,' I acknowledge curiously.

Nature always has a surprise in store.

# PARAKEET

───◊───

Right, so what's the point in this chapter? I hear you ask. Why have I spent so much time romanticising an invasive species? Why didn't I focus on some of the native species which live here in the UK? Instead I've dedicated time to a species that causes controversy, and I'm sure some people will complain about the inclusion of parakeets in a book about birds. But, the thing is, as I'm sure you've noticed by now, this isn't just a book about birds. It's actually a book about the silly, magical, curious joy that I feel when I see pretty much anything. It's a book about how connecting with the birds outside my front door has shown me how to deal with a lot of the turbulence that life throws at me and the lessons that have come along with that. It's a book that, I hope, will pass on that silly, magical, curious joy to you, so that next time you step out of your front door, or are fed up with the school run, you will notice that something new. Something that brings a new sense of delight, like a goose (or a duck) in an unexpected place. And once you do, you'll start to notice just how incredible the world becomes.

Parakeets, the non-native, screechy kites which stream through the skies of London and beyond, fill me with such excitement every time I see them – and that's what I'm trying to capture. That joy. Nothing on Earth is permanent. That – perhaps unfortunately, depending on how you look at it – is a fundamental truth that underpins the very fabric of our existence here on this planet.

From the highest mountain ranges to the tiniest microorganisms, everything is subject to the inevitability of time. Species dominate and fall – think dinosaurs – continents shift and even the stars will eventually fade away (there's some Oasis song lyrics in there somewhere). Nature reminds us of this impermanence in so many ways. The seasons change, each year bringing with them conditions which we mark as 'surprising' and 'unpredictable'. Rivers carve deep canyons through rock, eroding the Earth's foundations to create their own relentless paths. Even the tallest trees eventually succumb, returning to the soil that they came from. And that impermanence isn't limited to the natural world.

In our human world, we are all too aware that we are not here forever and perhaps this knowledge teaches us humility, reminding us that we are but fleeting specks in the grand tapestry of the cosmos. And so, as we navigate the ever-changing landscape of our lives, let us embrace the impermanence of all things. Let us find solace in the knowledge that, in the end, nothing lasts forever, and that our time on this Earth is but a brief and beautiful moment in the vast expanse of eternity.

The world is constantly moving, constantly changing; it's up to us humans whether or not we change with it.

# 12
# PIGEON

*'So long as men can breathe or eyes can see,
so long lives this, and this gives life to thee.'*
— Sonnet 18

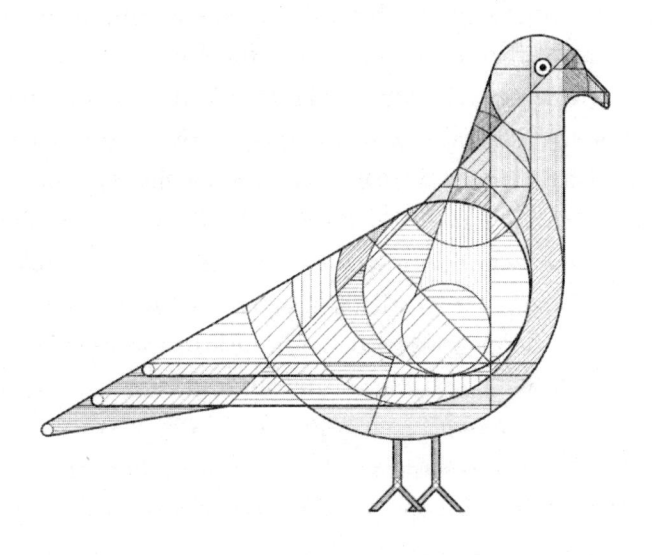

**Open your eyes now to the magic that surrounds you**

Every morning, if I've got the bedroom window open, one of the first sounds I am greeted by is the clattering of a wooden bird table falling on my patio as the resident wood pigeon, named Marlene by my kids, smashes against it in an awkward and undignified crash landing. And, every morning, as I look out of the window, she shakes herself off, unphased, and begins to pick through the seed that she has just scattered over the ground. I always think wood pigeons look a bit, well, stupid. They seem to have a glazed expression with not much going on behind the eyes. But get to know them and you'll realise they are funny characters with individual habits and personalities. And they're quite beautiful, with sturdy looking grey bodies, an almost blueish tinge in the right light and that pinky tint to the chest. I often think they look a bit like Mr Burns from *The Simpsons* with their large beaks. During spring, wood pigeons sing their chorus of *'be careful, Charlie'* (that's what I hear ever since Nick Acheson pointed out the sound and I stand by it) down the chimney-breast and tap-dance across the conservatory roof as they perform their courtship dances. While you might not notice them, I bet you see pigeons nearly every day. Whether you're in the middle of a city or in rural countryside, they are there. People will do their best to deter them from their garden feeders and cast them aside as 'just pigeons', but if you look a bit harder, open your eyes to the magic around you, hopefully, you'll see that pigeons, whether the city centre type or a wood pigeon, are really something quite spectacular. So much more than 'just a pigeon'.

———◊———

We have reached the final chapter, and 'Pigeon' is going to be either the easiest thing I've ever written or the most challenging.

You may be wondering why, after exploring eleven wonderful species which all have their unique stories to tell, I have chosen to conclude this book with the humble pigeon. The reason is simple: they're my favourite birds. 'What?' people often exclaim when I tell them that. But honestly, to me, there is no better species to capture the imagination and to act as an accessible gateway species in getting people more interested in nature. As with everything, there's so much more to pigeons than meets the eye and I'm going to do my best to help you fall in love with them, too – or at least appreciate them. So, please bear with me.

If you get off the boat that ferries you back and forth across Lake Windermere in the Lake District, you'll find yourself looking back across the largest lake in England at a view of the towering mountains that seem to frame the still water. Today, the blue sky is dotted with perfect clouds and looks a bit like a Windows XP screensaver. The drizzle that passed through has just about tailed off, leaving behind it a perfect, complete arching rainbow which paints vivid colours against the rugged backdrop of the high peaks. A Canada goose stands nearby, dipping its webbed toes in the water; it's considering taking the cold plunge and I bend down to take a photo of the scene, the goose perfectly framed by the rainbow. Nature's masterpiece.

The kids are starving so after a quick stop-off in a lakeside café, we pick up some duck food that's on sale at the counter, and head back out to see which birds are going to take up our offerings. George, my youngest, stands in his stripey blue and white rugby shirt, his messy hair tussling with the wind, and plunges his hand into the paper bag which contains the goods. Out of nowhere, a swan the same height as George appears and snaffles the food out of his hand. He laughs. 'Oh, I just fed a swan!' Not wanting to miss out on the fun, I take some food out of my own paper bag and offer it to the swan, which takes it, but I am soon joined by a perfectly white pigeon which lands on the sleeve of my fleece and begins to take food directly out of the open bag. I watch for a few minutes as the bird bravely continues to help itself, using me as a perch.

'I'm holding a pigeon,' George's voice sounds from behind me, amused. 'Argh, I'm holding three, help!' I turn around to see my son covered in pigeons, all helping themselves to his bag. They're lining up on his arms and shoulders while he stands like a scarecrow, laughing his little head off. I start to laugh and his brother, Jack, joins in, as does Mum, and before long we are crying with laughter at the scene in front of us. George, like some kind of urban Snow White or Mary Poppins feeding the birds.

So why am I so taken with birds that many people consider little more than vermin? Well, let's talk about pigeons, not shiny wood pigeons but feral pigeons or city pigeons, the ones you see in just about every town centre and car park, inside bins, sharing a curry that has been discarded on the ground or tugging at pieces of KFC chicken. These urban street pigeons are descendants of rock doves which you can still see nesting on Scottish and Irish coastlines. Their history intertwines with our own and stretches back thousands of years.

Rock doves were among the first birds that humans domesticated. The Egyptians, Persians and Greeks kept them for various purposes, including communication and as a source of food. Romans were particularly fond of pigeons, using them for messaging in the days of empire. Seems weird to imagine Romans using pigeons to pass messages between armies, pigeons helping the Romans to expand their empire, only to end up, millennia later, fighting in a wheelie bin over a Krispy Kreme.

Pigeons continued to play a significant role during wartime as messengers, carrying vital communications across enemy lines. Their remarkable homing ability and navigational skills made them invaluable assets in military operations, particularly during the First and Second World Wars. However, with the advent of modern communication technologies such as radio and, later, the internet, the use of pigeons as messengers declined sharply.

Like dogs, which are now a regular addition to human households and range in size and colour, the domestication process made rock doves more tolerant of humans and altered their behaviour, leading to the development of numerous pigeon breeds which varied in size, colour and plumage patterns. They served different functions such as racing, exhibition or meat production. Alongside domestication, some pigeons escaped or were released into the wild, gradually adapting to urban environments. These now feral pigeons found abundant food sources and shelter in cities, thriving in an anthropogenic landscape. As cities expanded and urbanisation accelerated, feral pigeon populations grew, establishing themselves worldwide as industrialisation rose, and the abundance of food scraps in city centres proved an ideal place for them to breed. Like herring gulls, parakeets and even peregrines, feral pigeons have adapted perfectly to urban life; they're just doing what they can to survive.

Are you ready for my favourite pigeon fact, the one that blew my mind when I found out? Pigeons produce milk. *What?* I hear you cry. *Milk!* How can birds produce milk? Okay, so they don't produce milk in the same way that mammals do, but they possess a unique adaptation known as 'crop milk' which allows both male and females to feed their young. Crop milk is a nutritious secretion (sounds tasty, doesn't it?), so named because it's produced in the 'crop', a specially evolved pocket at the base of the pigeon's throat.

The milk contains a rich blend of proteins, fats, carbohydrates, vitamins and minerals providing essential nutrients for the growth and development of pigeon chicks. Literally like baby formula – but for pigeons. This nutrient-rich substance allows pigeon parents to nourish their offspring even in environments where food sources may be scarce and even means that if the conditions are right, then pigeons don't have to wait for the breeding season and can reproduce at any time of the year. The only other birds able to produce this crop milk are flamingos and penguins, and everyone loves them! So, why not pigeons? I'm hoping this is a tick in the box for the 'pigeons are amazing' campaign. I think it's pretty cool that this adaptation allows them to successfully raise their young even in challenging environments.

I'm sitting on the sofa, my attention half on writing this chapter and half on a spreadsheet with a social media calendar that I'm planning for my current freelancing contract. I am always distracted by birds outside, and it comes as no surprise when I hear a knock-knock-knocking on the glass. Curious, I turn to look and spy a young pigeon perching on the windowsill, seemingly staring directly back at me. This bird isn't quite a weird squab (baby pigeon) sitting on a nest; it's clearly fledged successfully and is entering its teenage era, but it's still not quite a fully formed adult. Its beak looks too big for its face and the feathers are still straggly. It hasn't developed that trademark wood pigeon sleekness of Marlene, crash-landing on the bird table every day. I smile at the visitor; it slips and steadies itself awkwardly before fixing its eyes back on me.

'What do you want, strange bird?' I ask out loud, as though half expecting an answer.

The bird doesn't move and I am momentarily torn between returning to the spreadsheet and giving in to the intrigue of this unexpected interruption. I look back at the spreadsheet for a few minutes before glancing up to see the pigeon still looking through the window at me. Not going to lie, it's feeling a bit weird now. I'm not sure if this is a calming connection with the natural world, or something I should be concerned about. I put the laptop to one side and stand up to see if that scares off my onlooker. To my surprise, it doesn't flinch. You know when I said wood pigeons have nothing going on behind the eyes?

I kneel on the other sofa which sits underneath the window, the soft emerald velvet caving slightly as I put my weight on it and lean on the back to look at the pigeon. It slips again but this time, unable to catch itself, falls unceremoniously on to the lawn below. Looking dazed, it stands up after a second and walks across the grass and down the drive, before taking off and landing on a branch of a tree opposite my house, where it continues to stare.

*How bizarre*, I think, secretly delighted by the encounter.

———◊———

It's April 2024 and I've recently taken on a short freelance contract for a London-based network of food growers. This week, it's Good to Grow Week, which is when community gardens are encouraged to open their doors to the public and put on events to inspire people to get involved in local green spaces.

I've been sitting on the tube for fifty-six minutes of my life so far, having literally travelled the entire length of the Central line. My destination? A community allotment in East Acton. I alight the train at White City, a part of London I've never explored before, and head for Phoenix Farm. The phone map says it's a fourteen-minute walk so I begin in the right direction, away from the busy main road and crossing into a residential zone. Blocks of flats line either side of the road and people hurry along, looking down at their phones, as they expertly dodge each other. I stop and look at a pair of insect hotels that have been installed on a grassy verge surrounded by parked cars. A little reminder that there's still nature even here in this busy locale. I walk past the Queens Park Rangers' stadium, and as I round the corner, I see a brown sign indicating where I need to head. Turning down a narrow street which leads off from the main road, I walk towards a leisure centre tucked behind a row of houses until I spot the entrance to the garden. Walking through the gate, I am greeted by a huge space filled with plants of all shapes and sizes, trees where blue tits hop between the branches, and rows and rows of beds freshly raked and awaiting vegetables and fruits to be planted ahead of the new growing season. A wood pigeon wanders up and down one of the beds in the hope of finding some seeds to snack on, feet flicking up grains of soil with each step. A woman wearing khaki-coloured trousers and a bright pink T-shirt stops turning over soil as I walk up to her and introduce myself. I'm here with just one job: to see what activities they have on for Good to Grow Week and to take a few photos. She beckons me further into the garden where I see glasshouses full of plants, polytunnels, sheds and a communal area covered by a wooden pagoda where a few families sit reading children's books and colouring in images of birds and bugs.

The woman, Charlotte, invites me to take photos as she replants some nigella in a small trough. We chat as she works. Initially shy, she quickly warms to me and tells me she has volunteered at the community gardens for nine years and can't imagine not coming here a few times a week to work. Before she started at the garden, she knew very little about plants and growing food, but now she can't imagine her life without it. I wonder if she finds the garden peaceful; it seems it to me. As soon as I walked through the gate it was as if a soundproof force field went up blocking out the sound of the road and replacing it was a cawing corvid and a cooing wood pigeon.

'Do you find coming here is peaceful or relaxing?' I ask, expecting a similar answer to the one I receive from most other people I've spoken to who've discovered nature later in their lives.

'Nah, not really. You know, sometimes it's mega stressful trying to keep up with the planting and maintenance, relocating weeds, cleaning up,' she replies honestly and I'm a little taken aback by her response.

'What do you mean relocating weeds?' I pick up on her wording – usually people just say 'weeding'.

'A weed is a plant in the wrong place, so I just move them so they can grow somewhere else. Some of them are beautiful and they're still plants.' Shrugging, she sticks a nigella plant into a small hole she has just created.

What a refreshing attitude, one I should take on board in my own garden, though my current gardening knowledge and ability is embarrassingly lacking. 'Do you wish you'd found this garden earlier in your life?'

'Nope. I was just like the other kids in the area, I wasn't interested in gardening, or even being outside. I hung out with my mates and went to the gym and that. I think I would have laughed at someone who said they were into gardening. But as you grow up, people get their own lives and don't need the same personality as their friends anymore. You find your thing. Gardening is my thing now; maybe when I'm old I'll find a new thing, maybe do some travelling or something. But you find your thing when the time is right for you, I reckon.'

The matter of factness with which she says all this washes over me and I realise that perhaps, all this time, the regret I've felt for not reconnecting sooner with nature, with birds, is unfounded. Perhaps, it just wasn't the right time for me, and I needed to wait to find 'my thing'. As we chat, Charlotte gives me effortless hints and tips for my own garden, telling me about her own life and asking me about mine. Later, as I say goodbye, I am beaming from ear to ear, thinking about her words and the profound realisation she's triggered in me. I didn't do something wrong by not connecting with nature sooner; I just needed to wait until it found me, which I suppose is exactly what that oystercatcher did. It found me that day when I needed it the most.

After travelling all the way back east along the Central line to my next community garden in Bethnal Green, I have some time to kill so I wander to Victoria Park for lunch. I stand on the lake's edge watching a coot with two tiny fluffy babies squeaking away as they try to keep up with their mother. There are pedalos filled with families, dads with aching legs peddling their boats around the lake past me.

I smile as I walk past a couple arguing in a rowing boat. Both sit at one end of a small blue boat, which is sinking with the uneven weight, one end sticking up out of the water like a tiny *Titanic*.

'You need to move, I'm not going in this water with all the duck shit,' the woman hisses at her boyfriend, who begins to edge himself towards the other end of the boat, causing the whole thing to wobble dangerously.

I glance down at the tarmac to see a group of six feral pigeons unbothered by my presence. They're such fun to watch as they peck at the ground looking for food. A male, feathers all fluffed up, struts around, approaching every female like some annoying bloke in a bar trying it on with anyone. Each of the females in turn snub him, favouring the continued search for food.

A family stops next to me and begins to feed some bread to a swan which has waddled up to greet them. The two children smile and laugh as a few mallards wander over to see what all the fuss is about, and they are warmly welcomed by the family. The pigeons, having noticed that there is some food on offer, quickly hustle and, mimicking the ducks, wander about the family's feet. Almost immediately, the mood changes, the parents allowing the kids to kick out at the pigeons, scattering them as they anxiously take to the sky.

Regardless of the species, I wonder why any parent would allow their children to behave like that towards another living creature. What is it about pigeons that triggers such a negative reaction? Swans, ducks and pigeons are all birds, right? So why is one species considered to be less worthy of attention and celebration than others?

I wander into the café and grab a cheese croissant to eat before heading to my next garden. Sitting down on a bench by the lake, I am immediately joined by a pigeon landing next to me, boldly expecting a share of the croissant.

'I feed the pigeons, I sometimes feed the sparrows too / It gives me a sense of enormous well-being,' the voice of Phil Daniels in Blur's 'Parklife' pops into my head and I think they were on to something when they wrote those lyrics. I sprinkle a couple of crumbs and look at the bird. I don't think I've ever seen a brown pigeon. She's striking, with an iridescent blend of rose and emerald around her collar. Slender and elegant. If she were a rare bird with colours like that, birders and photographers would be rushing here to capture her image. She's really quite beautiful as she sits next to me, innocently going about her life, trying to survive every day in the city. But she's not rare; she's a pigeon. And perhaps I am the only person in the world to sit here and appreciate her. Part of me is saddened by that, but a large part of me feels privileged that I can marvel in her uniqueness. I just wish others would stop and notice her and the other individuals with their uniquely painted feathers, like fingerprints, each one different to the next.

'You've got cheese on your face!' The Yorkshire accent takes me by surprise, and I look up to see a man in a yellow fleece pointing at me. I quickly remove the cheese from the corner of my mouth, slightly embarrassed, and before I can utter a thank you, he sprinkles a couple of crumbs from his own sandwich on to the bench for the pigeon still perched next to me, before walking away. Perhaps I'm not alone after all.

I carry on through the park, exploring the vast green space that sprawls in front of me. Wildflower verges, ornate gardens, huge playing fields, a diverse and glorious space hiding among the houses, shops and tower blocks, unsuspecting, but warmly welcome in the fog of chaos that dictates our day to day lives.

I pass picnicking families, a sports pavilion where a group of lads are working out on the outdoor gym equipment, a tennis court with two games in play, a couple with binoculars around their necks, a football match on the large flat field. I look around and see the park is framed by tall trees which seem to block it off and protect us all from the busy city that lies in wait beyond the thick trunks. It's a Saturday afternoon and in London all of these people could be doing anything. Shopping, the theatre, art galleries, museums, exhibitions, bars, restaurants, London is a city of endless possibilities; there's always something to do. And yet, here are all of these people sharing this green space. There's so much choice and still these people have gathered here to spend their day off.

Whether the people around me are consciously connecting with the nature that surrounds them or not, they're here playing football as the starlings forage in the grass, picnicking alongside the pigeons. It strikes me that most people have an innate drive to get outside as often as they can. Whether it's a lunchtime stroll to get some fresh air or heading out to look at a rare bird, people choose to step outside. During the COVID-19 pandemic, there was an increase in people spending time in green spaces when we were allowed to, admitting that we felt better for the time outside. A lot of us found ourselves suddenly with more free time than we were used to; we used that time to get out.

The Mental Health Foundation produced a report that stated 45 per cent of people admitted that connecting with nature in some way, be it walking, listening to birdsong or gardening, helped them through the pandemic. Some 73 per cent of adults said connecting with nature was vital for management of their mental health; 65 per cent of people stated that they felt a flood of positive emotion when spending time doing something 'naturey'. So, most of us do feel better being outside.

By 2050, it's estimated that around 70 per cent of people in the world will be living in urban areas as we continue on our path of 'world domination', and 25 per cent of young adults feel they are not able to connect with nature in the way they would like as they don't feel safe. Yet nature is good for us. Like, *really* good for us. If nothing else encourages you to connect, if the plight of the curlew doesn't fill you with sadness, if you don't feel regret over the loss of swifts from our skies, if you don't feel compelled to connect with nature to save it, how about connecting with it in order to save yourself? By definition, if we at least do that, if everyone starts feeling the benefit of this free therapy tool, then we will surely automatically want to protect it.

If we have to mobilise people through their selfishness, then so be it. But I'm full of hope and I have more faith than that in humans. Nature is good for us, and we can be good for nature. After all, it's part of us and we are part of it. We are as much nature as the ethereal, elemental swifts. We are as much part of it as the feral pigeons on the South Bank.

Embrace that knowledge, hold on to it and be part of it. Let it fill your existence.

We have built up these concrete jungles around us, and now it feels as if we are on a desperate mission to create green spaces within them to counteract what we have done and give us the opportunity to reconnect with our wild roots. A cyclist glides past me; she could have got a taxi. A man sits on a bench with a boombox blasting out rap; he could be sitting inside his flat listening to the music. Whether we are up a Welsh mountain seeking the solitude it offers, photographing gannets on a cliff, feeding pigeons on a dirty bench in Victoria Park – if we realise it or not, we each have moments every single day where we connect with nature in one way or another. The sooner we embrace that fact, then the sooner we can start working towards a future where we live in harmony with the natural world.

I set out to write this book with two aims. The first to show you that there is beauty to be found in every corner and crevice. Whether you are in the middle of a busy city centre or on a rural coastline, there is something wonderful waiting for you. And I hope that by taking you back on a time-travelling trip through my memories, my journey into nature and the birds I love, I have managed to do that. My second aim wasn't to do with nature at all. It was to do with you. I wanted to share with you the twelve lessons that I have learnt over the last couple of years as I've reconnected with nature, and by doing so show you how nature has helped me to navigate my everyday life, dealing with the most mundane problems as well as the bigger stuff that can sometimes seem impossible to survive. I wanted to share with you the magical gifts and life lessons that I have been offered through spending time immersing myself in nature, particularly with birds.

Writing this book has allowed me a lot of time to reflect on the past couple of years, and I realise how lucky I am to have encountered so many people who have, often unknowingly, guided me towards this path. Francis Hickenbottom, my physics teacher, didn't set out that day to show me the peregrines; he didn't know that one day I would be unable to see a cathedral spire without casting my eyes to the sky in search of these birds. Alex Georgiev didn't know that, during our walk in Bangor, he would reveal to me a natural symphony that surrounds us every day, like he was handing over a playlist packed full of songs that I'd never heard before. Sean McCormack doesn't know how, by showing me a glimpse of the nature in Ealing, he opened up my eyes to a world of urban wildlife that I never knew was there before. Hannah Bourne-Taylor doesn't know that her passion and dedication to a particular species of bird fills me with hope and confidence that maybe, just maybe, we can make a positive change. All of these people, in fact everyone mentioned in this book, are likely unaware of the impact they have had on my life, and how they directed me on to my journey of self-discovery.

The Earth is at a pivotal moment where we need to start hearing each other in order to ensure that the beauty and wonder that is all around us is able to continue to thrive as we hurtle deeper and deeper into an anthropogenic world. We need to use our uniquely human abilities to share with each other the magic that surrounds us every day. Storytelling makes us human, so why don't we take the opportunity to share our knowledge with each other? We have the power to travel to the moon, the ability to put roving machines on other planets and search for traces of life that may or may not have once existed. We can do anything. So now, I think it's about time we start paying attention not to distant galaxies, but to the stars that twinkle here right on our own doorsteps. To the treasure that lies in wait just outside our front doors, in our trees and skies. It's as easy as just taking the time to look at stuff. *See* it. It might turn out to be a squashed berry on the path, a twig sticking out of a hedgerow or a plastic bag blowing in the breeze. On the other hand, it could turn out to be something rather marvellous.

So now, all that is left to do is hand over the pair of magic glasses that were given to me by everyone I have encountered on my journey. I don't need them anymore, I can see without them, so I'm giving them to you in the hope that you will put down this book, put them on and allow them to help you adjust your focus. To start seeing the wonders that are, quite literally, everywhere. Appreciate the unique beauty of everything you encounter: a pigeon, an oystercatcher, a curlew, a rook. Notice nature, let it in and, I promise you, your world will become truly magnificent.

Open your eyes to the treasures that surround you and experience the life-affirming magic of birds.

### Special thanks to:

Jules Bingham
Nick Acheson
Lev Parikian
Chet Cuñago
Hannah Bourne-Taylor
Dr Sean McCormack
Simon Beedie
Megan Shersby
Dan Rouse
Ryan Dalton
Rory Dimond
Connor Alves
Francis Hickenbottom
Dr Alexander Georgiev
Stephen Moss
Robin Ince
Amberley Lowis
Chris Stone
Cromer Peregrine Project

Sam Viles
Ptolemy McKinnon
Hope Robson
Elaine Payne
Yoav Perlman
Mark Rosen
Lottie Glover
Kyle Heesom
Sarah Cunningham
Sue and John Beckwith
Matt Spracklen
Bryony Moss
Lu Stanton-Greenwood
Giselle Rainsford-Betts
Natalie and John White
Jon Staples
Kate McCrae
Professor Ben Garrod

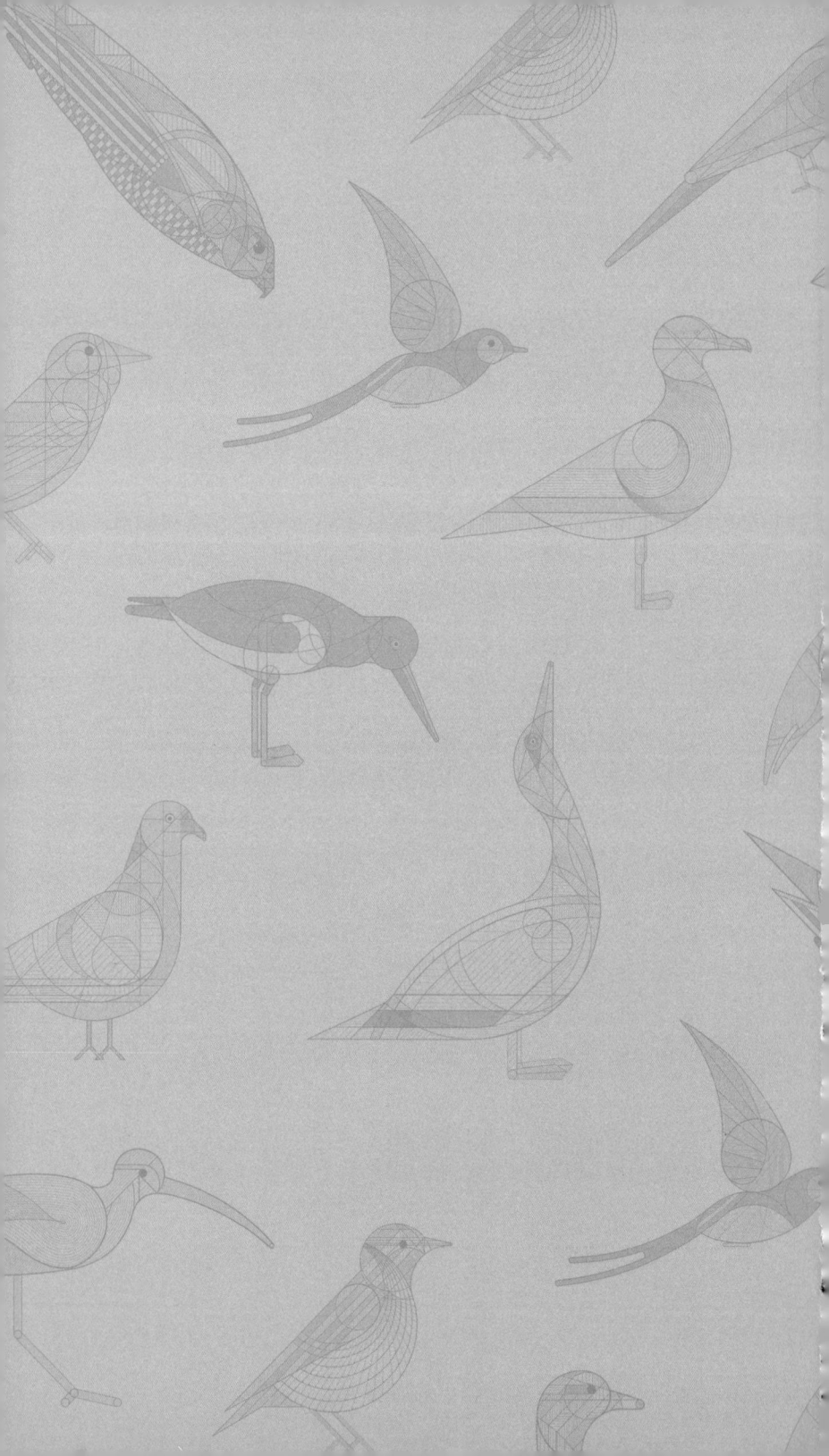